AF342530

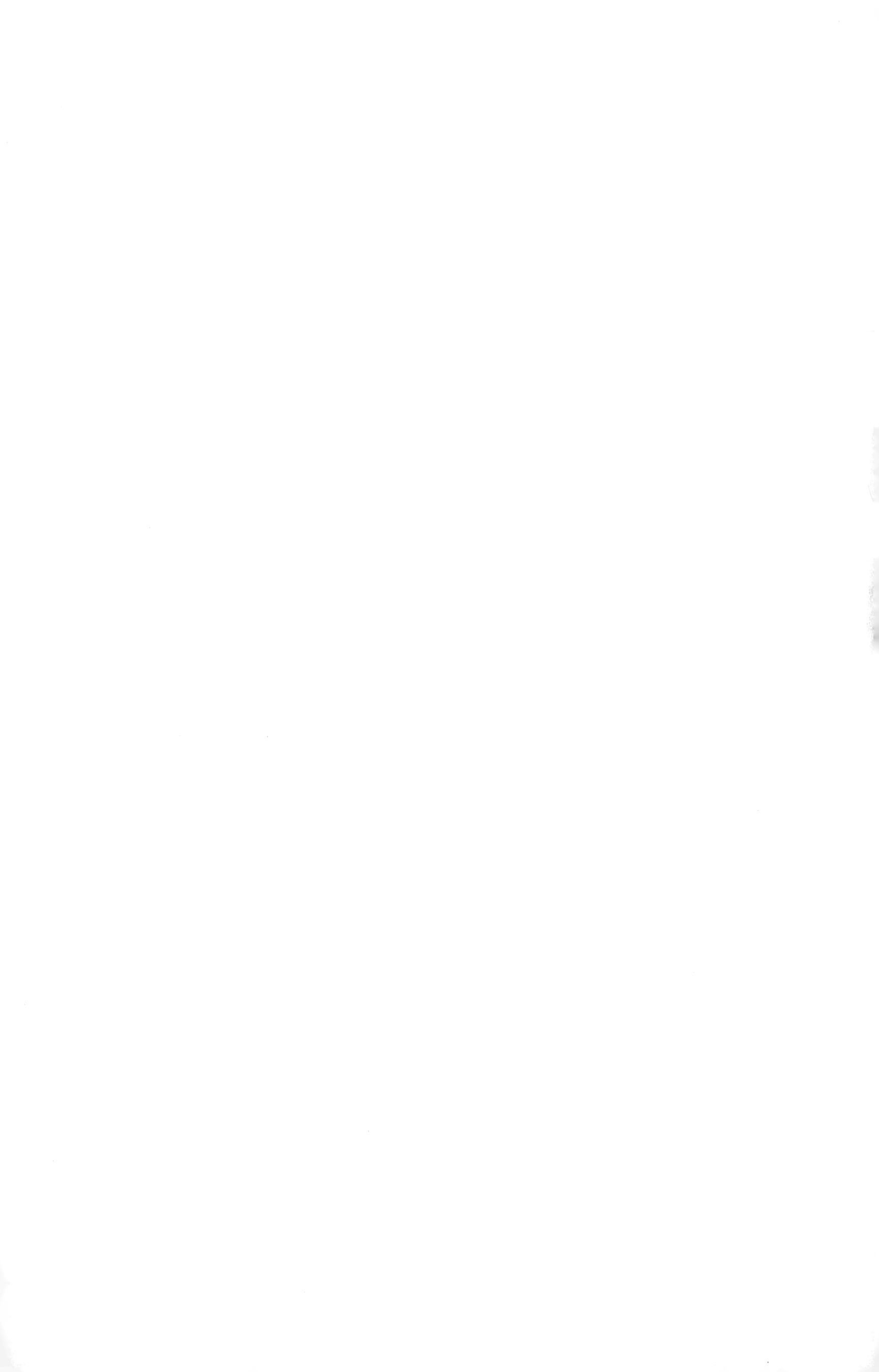

NEW DEVELOPMENTS IN MEDICAL RESEARCH

CRYOSURGERY AND COLPOSCOPY

PRACTICES, OUTCOMES AND POTENTIAL COMPLICATIONS

LILLIAN WATSON
EDITOR

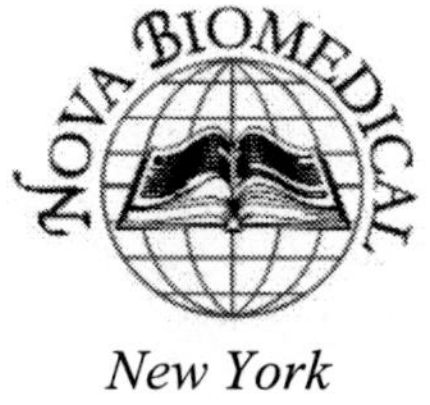

Nova Biomedical

New York

NOTICE TO THE READER

Library of Congress Cataloging-in-Publication Data

Library of Congress Control Number: 2015960467

ISBN: 978-1-63484-507-6

Published by Nova Science Publishers, Inc. † New York

CONTENTS

Contents

PREFACE

Cryosurgery is a common procedure, known for thousands of years. Cryoablation causes tissue necrosis by freezing the targeted tissues. Necrosis results from the freezing and thawing of cells (crystallization water) and the sequestration of the dead tissue by the organism. After removal of the lesion, regeneration through the layering of a new epithelium starts. Cryosurgery is a safe procedure which does not cause pain or bleeding. It may be performed in an outpatient clinic and premedication is not necessary. The first section of this book focuses on cryosurgery.

Chapter 1 – Cryosurgery is a common procedure, known for thousands of years. The use of low temperatures dates back to the ancient Egyptians. Later Hippocrates recommended the use of cold as an analgesic, to reduce edema and control bleeding. In otolaryngology, cryosurgery is applied in the following diseases: epistaxis, nasal mucosal hemangiomas (hemangiomas, "bleeding polyp" of the nasal septum, pyogenic granuloma), chronic hypertrophic rhinitis – including allergic and non-allergic rhinitis, precancerous conditions of the nose (papillomas, leukoplakia), malignant tumors (early limited cancerous changes of the nasal skin or mucous membrane in stage T1N0M0) and also diseases of the oral cavity and larynx. The use of cryosurgery in patients with both allergic and non-allergic rhinitis is worth noting as it is an alternative to not always effective pharmacotherapy. It is recommended for patients in whom conventional therapy was not satisfactory. Cryoablation causes tissue necrosis by freezing the targeted tissues. Necrosis results from the freezing and thawing of cells (crystallization water) and the sequestration of the dead tissue by the organism. After removal of the lesion, regeneration through the layering of a new epithelium starts. Cryosurgery is a safe procedure which does not cause pain or bleeding. It may be performed in an outpatient clinic and premedication is not necessary. Our studies on patients with both allergic and non-allergic rhinitis showed statistically significant improvement in subjective evaluation of nasal obstruction, which was also observed on rhinomanometric examination. On endoscopic examination, 63.3% patients with allergic rhinitis and 76.7% patients with non-allergic rhinitis showed improvement in nasal obstruction which lasted 3-4 months. Cryosurgery is not the treatment of first choice as it does not remove the cause of the disease, however, it significantly improves the quality of life in patients with allergic and non-allergic rhinitis in combination with other methods.

Chapter 2 – The percentages of incidentally discovered renal cell carcinoma (RCC) has increased recently due to the routine use of cross-sectional imaging in the diagnosis and follow up of different diseases. More than 50% of incidentally discovered RCCs are diagnosed in patients with advanced age, which is an age group associated with multiple co-morbidities. Luckily, most RCCs are incidentally discovered at a very early stage (Stage 1A). The combination of early stage disease and multiple co-morbidities favored nephron sparing minimal invasive surgeries, such as ablation techniques. Cryosurgery plays an important role in the management of these patients and became one of the standard of care options for management of stage 1A RCC. When performed either percutaneously or laparoscopically, cryosurgery is considered the most frequently used ablative technique in management of RCC. Furthermore, cryosurgery has been well reported in the management of other non-RCC renal tumors.

Chapter 3 – Colposcopy is an important device or method in the diagnosis of cervical lesions and prevention of cervical cancer. Cervical cancer screening programs can be divided into three basic points: screening, management of abnormal cytology and management in post-treatment. Cervical intraepithelial neoplasia is defined by cellular atypia confined to the epithelium. The screening of these lesions is performed by Pap's smear. This method has good sensitivity and high specificity, but there is criticism because the rates of false-negative results (10-30%) due to limitations of the procedure. Colposcopy is performed in abnormal cervical cytology. The sensitivity of the test is 85%-96% and specificity around 48%-69%. The specificity and predictive positive value for CIN 2/3 and invasive carcinoma is around 83% and 71.8%, respectively. Colposcopic imaging must evaluate the following parameters: acetowhitening kinetics, vascular pattern and Lugol iodine solution staining (Schiller Test). According to the gradation of the displayed signals, it is estimated the degree of commitment by the injury. Biopsy must be addressed in places where alterations are viewed for definitive diagnosis.

Less than 1% of Pap smear results are diagnosed as atypical glandular cells. These findings are divided by Bethesda System in Atypical Glandular cells of undetermined significance (AGC), adenocarcinoma in situ and invasive adenocarcinoma of uterine cervix. The initial conduct for these patients is very variable and include colposcopy with directed biopsy, endocervical and endometrial curettage. The research of HPV DNA also has an essential role, especially in cases of AGC, which often have significant correlation with clinically important lesions, including invasive adenocarcinoma, identifying those with a higher risk of injury.

In post-treatment, colposcopy is important for monitoring recurrent disease. The main objective of CIN 2/3 excisional treatment is the complete removal of the lesion and transformation zone, leading to a proper interpretation of the margins by the pathologist. The margins status can predict the risk of recurrent disease. The decision of retreatment depends on follow-up with cytology and colposcopy, and some current protocols add HPV biomolecular testing. Advances in the understanding of cervical carcinogenesis and their relation with the human papillomavirus (HPV) has led to new prevention strategies based on HPV testing. Still, colposcopy remains an important method in the initial evaluation of patients with positive high-risk HPV testing, and realization of cervical biopsy.

The aim of this chapter is to address the different colposcopic findings in squamous and glandular cervical lesions, and demonstrate the performance of colposcopy in cervical intraepithelial lesions diagnosis.

Chapter 4 – Vaginal Intraepithelial Neoplasia (VaIN) is a rare preinvasive disease that accounts for up to 1% of women who attend the colposcopy clinic. In this chapter the authors will review the characteristics of the disease (i.e., location in the vagina, single versus multifocal presentation), the risk factors for VaIN (i.e., other invasive or pre-invasive disease of the low genital tract, smoking), methods of screening for the diagnosis (including vaginal cytology, oncHPV testing), and role of colposcopy in making the diagnosis. Strategies for enhancing the colposcopic identification of VaIN will be discussed such as the use of vaginal estrogen, use of 3-5% acetic acid and Lugol's solution.

Treatment strategies, indications for specific maneuvers and the likelihood of success and complications will be presented for 5FU (Effudex®), CO_2 laser ablation/excision, upper vaginectomy, colpectomy, vaginal brachytherapy, and Aldara®. Recommendations for follow-up will be provided.

Chapter 5 – Cervical dysplasia diagnosed at or before hysterectomy or recent dyskaryosis on a cervical smear are considered risk factors for the development of vaginal intraepithelial neoplasia (VaIN) following hysterectomy. Current guidance recommends vault cytology in women who are at increased risk of VaIN but evidence of benefit is weak. This is a retrospective cohort study of 330 women who had a hysterectomy for benign pathology. The follow up practice and the results of vaginal pathology were recorded 24 and 60 months following surgery. One case of high grade vaginal intraepithelial neoplasia was recorded but no cases of vaginal cancer were diagnosed in the high risk group of patients within a 5 year period post hysterectomy. Relevant studies predate routine human papilloma virus (HPV) testing and there is limited data regarding the course of vaginal HPV infections in the absence of a cervix. The available evidence is reviewed and an approach for the follow up of this group of women is suggested.

Chapter 6 – Postcoital bleeding (PCB) is defined as spotting or bleeding that occurs during or after sexual intercourse unrelated to menstruation. It is a common gynecological symptom and is often alarming for women. The point prevalence of PCB determined in large community surveys ranges from 0.7 to 9% with an annual cumulative incidence of around 6% of menstruating women. Up to 5% of women are seen in a hospital's gynecology outpatient department due to PCB.

PCB could be the first sign of serious underlying pathology such as cervical intra-epithelial neoplasia (CIN), cervical carcinoma or chlamydial infection. It is estimated that the prevalence of cervical carcinoma and CIN in women with PCB varied between 0%-8% and 6.8%-19% respectively. It was reported that all symptomatic women with cervical carcinoma under 65 years of age had PCB. Moreover, PCB was found in 18%-38.3% of chlamydia-positive women.

There is a great deal of controversy between gynecologists as regards managing women with PCB; probably due to the lack of well-designed studies and due to the variations in study design, including differences in symptom definition, time range in which the symptom occurred, frequency, age distribution of the population, and prevalence of sexually transmitted infection and use of hormones. Currently there are no well-defined guidelines available regarding how and where to manage these women. Many authors and experts recommend assessing women with PCB in the colposcopy clinic. However, other authors believe that, despite the well-reported association with serious pathology, referring every case of PCB for immediate investigation is inappropriate, impractical and not cost effective. This chapter will critically review the causes, risk factors and management of PCB in an attempt to outline a unified guidance based on the best available evidence for women and gynecologists alike.

Chapter 7 – The number of the patient with dysplasia and CIS of the uterine cervix has been increasing recently, especially in the younger ages who need fertility preservation. Although cervical conization is standard therapy for dysplasia and CIS, the significant increase in the obstetrical risks such as premature delivery after conization has been reported. On the other hand, PDT is an excellent procedure to treat dysplasia and CIS by photochemical reaction generated by laser irradiation to the lesion under colposcopy after injection of tumor-specific photosensitizer. The authors have developed protocol and colposcope specifically designed to PDT, and applied PDT to dysplasia and CIS for 20 years. PDT was performed for 520 cases (146 dysplasia, 342 CIS, 4 AIS, 24 MIC, 1 MIAC, 2 invasive SCC, and 1 invasive adenoca.). 97% (503/520) of PDT cases were CR by the first PDT. 8 out of 16 PR cases turned out to be CR by the second PDT. CR rates for dysplasia, CIS, MIC were 99%, 97%, and 92%, respectively. These data suggest that PDT using colposcopy enables accurate LASER irradiation to uterine cervix resulting in high cure rate for CIN and early stage cervical cancer, and PDT for CIN and early stage uterine cervical cancer could be one of modalities of uterine preservation therapy as well as endocervical conization.

Chapter 8 – In the attempt to colposcopically examine the vulva, it is essential to know the histology of vulvar skin, since the complexity of the vulvar anatomy requires a different assessment of the seemingly same types of lesions in this area. Thickness of the vulvar skin affects the opacity; the vascular patterns are less marked and less marked and less reliable than with colposcopy of the cervix. Vascular aberrations, such as punctuations and mosaic, can be practically seen only on the inner portions of the labia minora where the keratin layer is thinner and vestibular epithelium does not contain a keratin layer.

SECTION ONE: CRYOSURGERY

Chapter 1

THE USE OF CRYOSURGERY IN OTOLARYNGOLOGY

Hanna Zielinska-Blizniewska[1,2] and Jurek Olszewski[2]

[1]Department of Allergology and Respiratory Rehabilitation,
Medical University of Lodz, Lodz, Poland
[2]Department of Otolaryngology, Laryngological Oncology,
Audiology and Phoniatrics, Medical University of Lodz, Lodz, Poland

ABSTRACT

Cryosurgery is a common procedure, known for thousands of years. The use of low temperatures dates back to the ancient Egyptians. Later Hippocrates recommended the use of cold as an analgesic, to reduce edema and control bleeding. In otolaryngology, cryosurgery is applied in the following diseases: epistaxis, nasal mucosal hemangiomas (hemangiomas, "bleeding polyp" of the nasal septum, pyogenic granuloma), chronic hypertrophic rhinitis – including allergic and non-allergic rhinitis, precancerous conditions of the nose (papillomas, leukoplakia), malignant tumors (early limited cancerous changes of the nasal skin or mucous membrane in stage T1N0M0) and also diseases of the oral cavity and larynx. The use of cryosurgery in patients with both allergic and non-allergic rhinitis is worth noting as it is an alternative to not always effective pharmacotherapy. It is recommended for patients in whom conventional therapy was not satisfactory. Cryoablation causes tissue necrosis by freezing the targeted tissues. Necrosis results from the freezing and thawing of cells (crystallization water) and the sequestration of the dead tissue by the organism. After removal of the lesion, regeneration through the layering of a new epithelium starts. Cryosurgery is a safe procedure which does not cause pain or bleeding. It may be performed in an outpatient clinic and premedication is not necessary. Our studies on patients with both allergic and non-allergic rhinitis showed statistically significant improvement in subjective evaluation of nasal obstruction, which was also observed on rhinomanometric examination. On endoscopic examination, 63.3% patients with allergic rhinitis and 76.7% patients with non-allergic rhinitis showed improvement in nasal obstruction which lasted 3-4 months. Cryosurgery is not the treatment of first choice as it does not remove the cause of the disease, however, it significantly improves the quality of life in patients with allergic and non-allergic rhinitis in combination with other methods.

HISTORY OF CRYOSURGERY

Cryosurgery is a common treatment, and one of the oldest. Medical use of low temperatures dates back to ancient Egypt. Hippocrates (460-377 BC) recommended low temperature as a local analgesic to reduce edema and bleeding [1]. In modern times Bartholinus (1616-1680) described medical use of ice and snow ("De nivis uso medico," 1661). In 1845 Arnott, considered the father of modern cryosurgery, described the benefits of local applications of cold for the treatment of many illnesses, mainly chronic headaches and neuralgia. He was a pioneer of the use of cryotherapy in oncology using salt solutions containing crashed ice at -18 to -24°C to not only decrease the size of tumors in breast cancer or cervical carcinoma but also to act as an analgesic. Arnott is also considered a pioneer of anesthesia by cooling. In 1847, Flaurens described analgesic properties of ethyl chloride used superficially. In patients, it was not used in the form of aerosol until 1866. Evaporation of ethyl chloride on the skin lowers its temperature to -15—20°C. Until now its anesthetic properties have been used mainly after contusions in sports medicine [1, 2, 3].

The beginnings of modern cryomedicine date back to the close of the 19th century, when physicists learned how to liquefy gas. In 1877 Cailletet (1832-1913) in France and Pictet (1846-1929) in Switzerland achieved the temperature of about 90K (-183°C) for a few seconds and observed liquefied oxygen in the form of a mist. In 1883, in Cracow, Polish scientists Olszewski (1846-1915) and Wroblewski (1845-1888) were the first in the world to liquefy oxygen, nitrogen and carbon dioxide from the atmosphere in a stable state. They obtained cryogenic liquids in large amounts so that they could describe fundamental physical constants and observe meniscus [1-4].

The era of cryogenic industry started in 1895 when Carl von Linde (1842-1932) produced large amounts of liquid air and distilled the air. The gifted inventor, the first producer of oxygen and nitrogen, became a successful entrepreneur. In 1907 Whitehouse constructed the first liquid nitrogen withdrawal device and used it to destroy superficially localized tumors and also to treat some of the dermatological diseases [5, 9].

From 1908 until the 1950s cryogenics developed in scientific laboratories, becoming a widely used tool for materials science. In the 1950s cryogenics discoveries started to be used in the production of heavy water, the cooling of superconductors, and the rocket and nuclear industries. Since 1961 a closed-cycle cooling system for applicators has been used. Gradually, copper and silver-metal probes were introduced. This resulted in the increased use of low temperatures in medicine, in both local and general cryotherapy [1].

Cryosurgery is the local, controlled use of extreme cold to destroy living cells. Cryotherapy is a stimulus-control treatment using local or general nondestructive activity of low temperatures.

MECHANISM OF ACTION

Studies on the mechanism of tissue destruction following freezing involve physical, chemical and biological phenomena explained by different theories. The mechanism of destruction of pathologically changed tissues is necrosis, which results from the freezing and thawing of cells, and is followed by the sequestration of the dead tissues by the organism. The treated area reepithelializes. Adverse effects (hyperemia and pain) are usually minor and short-lived. To achieve hypothermia, compressed gas under high pressure (mostly nitrous oxide, carbon dioxide or a special gas mixture) is forced through a small aperture in the probe. Cryoprobe coating is cooled due to the Joule-Thomson effect [5, 6].

Within a few seconds an extremely low temperature is achieved (-65°C – -85°C). The temperature of cell death is -20°C – -30°C [6]. Water crystallization is the most important phenomenon during tissue cooling. During freezing, intracellular fluid undergoes crystallization. Ice crystals destroy intracellular organella. The denaturation of proteins by intracellular dehydration follows on the cell membrane.

The tissue is also damaged by the cessation of blood flow and its stagnation in the microvasculature. Cell metabolism is inhibited after its cytoplasm freezing and thawing.

Sensitivity to cryotherapy is directly related to water content in tissues; the higher the water content, the greater the sensitivity to the therapy. Nose and throat tissues are a good area for the use of this therapeutic method. At low temperatures, extra- and intracellular ice cubes are formed in nasal mucosa. Water is removed from the cell. Osmotic pressure rises. Ph drops to level 4, which affects intracellular metabolism. After tissue necrosis caused by low temperatures and the removal of the pathological lesion, regeneration through the layering of a healthy epithelium starts. Initially the epithelium contains a large number of goblet cells followed by a ciliated pseudostratified columnar epithelium. The renewal lasts about 30 days. No scars or fibrosis are observed. Freezing also results in ice cube formation in venal, arterial and capillary blood vessels, which leads to ischemia and necrosis [5, 6].

EQUIPMENT

Laryngology specificity requires special equipment. Cryoprobes, basic tools, should have a diameter that allows endoscopy. The temperature of the outside surface depends on the thermal conductivity of the material used. Silver and copper are the best materials as they easily conduct the cold and effectively induce cell necrosis. The size of the necrosis depends on the cryoprobe contact with the lesion to be removed. The whole lesion should be covered by a cryoprobe tip. Cryoprobe may be covered with aqueous cream to impede the probe stick to mucosa [7].

Cryoapplicators in the shape of a needle, spatula, cone or cylinder may be used. We use mainly a spatula-shaped cryoprobe (Figure 1, Figure 2).

INDICATIONS FOR CRYOSURGERY IN OTORHINOLARYNGOLOGY

Miszka [8] and Moszynski [9] worked out indications for cryotherapy for the following otolaryngological conditions:

I   Diseases of the nose
1.   Persistent epistaxis (nose bleeds)
– bleeding from the nasal septum within Kisselbach's plexus,
– bleeding from the inferior nasal turbinate,
– bleeding from the posterior nasal cavity.

Hicks and Norris [10] studied 450 patients treated for epistaxis with cryotherapy. They found cryotherapy significantly superior to traditional methods: argentum nitricum, coagulation, nasal packing.

2.   Nasal mucosal hemangiomas
– haemangiomas,
– "bleeding polyp" of the nasal septum,
– pyogenic granuloma in the nasal cavity,
– Osler-Weber-Rendu disease (OWRD).

According to Moszynski and Miszka [9], cryosurgery is the treatment of choice for bleeding granuloma of the nasal septum, hemangiomas in the nasal cavity in the course of OWRD.

3.   Chronic rhinitis
– chronic hypertrophic rhinitis,
– chronic vasomotor rhinitis,
– allergic rhinitis.
4.   Precancerous conditions
– nasal papillomas,
– leukoplakia.
5.   Carcinomas
– limited neoplasia of the skin of the nose or mucosa T1N0M0.
II   Diseases of the pharynx
– chronic hypertrophic tonsillitis.

Chronic hypertrophic tonsillitis responds well to cryosurgery. The method involves a fast and deep tonsil freeze followed by the aspiration of the frozen tissue. The procedure may be done under local anesthesia. Hill [11] recommends nitrous oxide (-196°C). For tonsil freezing 2-3 applications for 3-4 min are indicated.

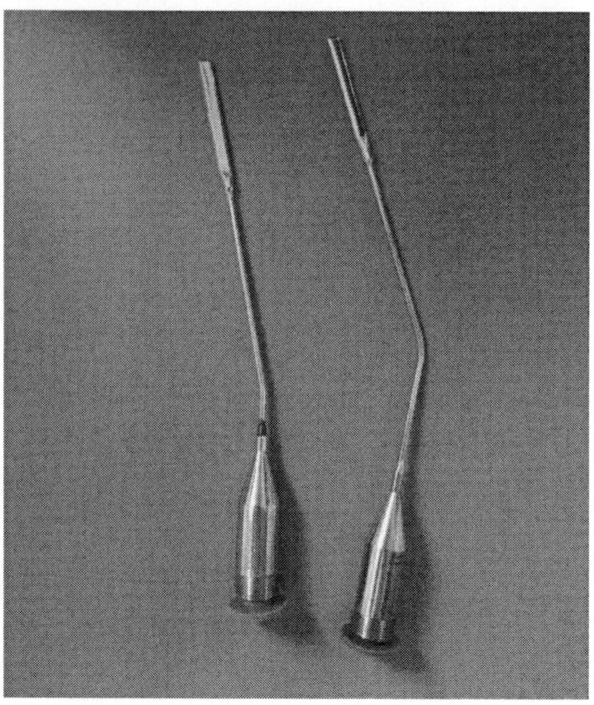

Figure 1. Cryoprobes.

Necrosis of the hypertrophic tissue and its tearing off the basis follows; the frozen tissue is then removed by aspiration. There is no significant bleeding due to endovascular thrombosis. During freezing, the pain is minor. The lymphoid tissue is not completely removed but the remnants are more resistant to infections. Cryosurgery inhibits the inflammatory process and leads to full anatomical and functional recovery.

III   Chronic diseases of the larynx
- childhood type papillomas,
- precancerous conditions (leukoplakia and pachydermia),
- post intubational granuloma,
- mucosal angiomas

Now, cryosurgery has been replaced by laser surgery in treating laryngeal diseases [7].

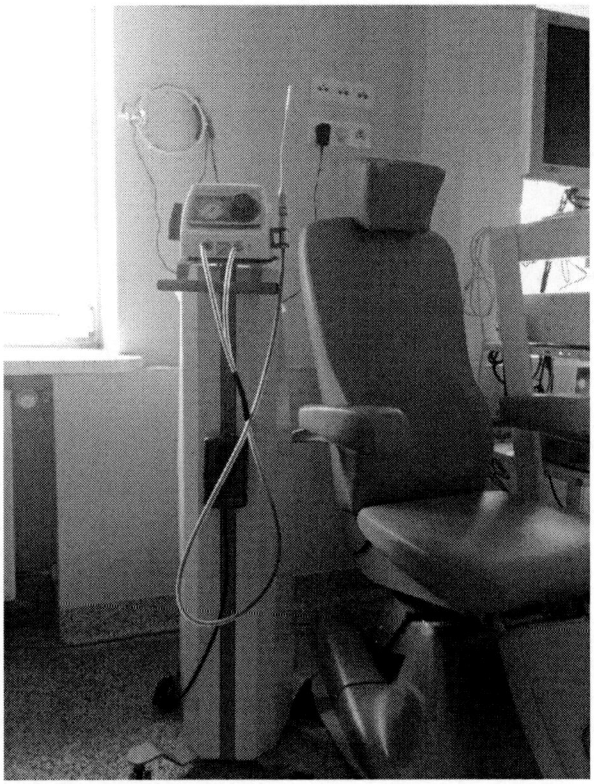

Figure 2. Set-up of cryoprobe in the office.

IV Other
1. Trigeminal neuralgia.

Zakrzewska [12] used decompression, thermocoagulation and cryotherapy to analyze long-term results of trigeminal neuralgia treatment. She found that full remission lasted over 5 years in 62% patients after decompression, 2 years after thermocoagulation and 6 months after cryotherapy.

In case of recurrence, cryoprobe is indicated to be placed on the same site as during the first procedure [12].

2. Snoring.

Snoring is an unpleasant symptom related to amyotonia of the soft palate. Nonactive muscle may be stimulated by cryotherapy.

A few short sessions, each 1-2 min, are required [5]. The use of cryosurgery in patients with rhinitis, both allergic and non- allergic, is noteworthy. It is an alternative to not always effective pharmacotherapy. It is recommended for patients for whom conventional treatment has not been satisfactory.

CRYOSURGERY IN CHRONIC RHINITIS

Pharmacological treatment of chronic rhinitis is not always effective. It refers particularly to non allergic and allergic rhinitis.

Non-allergic rhinitis refers to inflammation of nasal mucosa without a known cause, when allergic etiology cannot be confirmed. Skin tests are negative, total IgE is at norm, there is no allergen-specific IgE [13].

The underlying changes in both allergic and non-allergic rhinitis are due to hyperreactivity of nasal mucosa. Hyperreactivity may result from many conditions, e.g., epithelium damage, increased irritability of receptors in the nasal mucosa, changes in nerve conduction in the peripheral nervous system, mediator release and inflammatory cell infiltration [5].

Symptoms of allergic and non-allergic rhinitis are observed all year round, however, they increase in autumn and winter, mostly in the morning. Nasal congestion is the main symptom. Patients also complain of headaches, dry throat, particularly after the night, and discomfort. Due to chronic symptoms, both allergic and non-allergic rhinitis is a tiresome disease which involves the constant use of pharmaceuticals: both local and general.

Because they are not always effective, alternative therapies are necessary. Cryosurgery is one of them. Since 2006, cryoablation of nasal inferior conchae in patients with allergic and non-allergic rhinitis has been performed in the Department of Otolaryngology, Laryngologial Oncology, Audiology and Phoniatrics, Medical University of Lodz. Patients with no changes in the paranasal sinuses, diagnosed by CT, are qualified for the therapy. CT shows only edema and hypertrophy of the nasal inferior turbinates.

TECHNIQUE OF SURGERY

Cryosurgery is performed with the patient in a seated position and under local anesthesia of nasal mucosa (Lignocaine 4%, spray).

A nasal applicator is applied to the medial and inferior medial surface of the nasal inferior concha. The procedure is performed on both sides.

A single freeze lasts about 30 sec and is repeated 3 times. The procedure may be repeated after 3 months if the improvement is not satisfactory.

Cryosurgery is a safe and painless procedure that produces only minor bleeding. It may be performed in an outpatient clinic and does not require premedication.

DISCUSSION

Cryosurgery has advantages over electrocoagulation as the procedure is painless, leads to destruction of superficial tissue and does not destroy deeper structures. A superficially damaged epithelium regenerates.

Krecicki [7] showed that ciliary epithelium also regenerated and the resulting scars were thin and did not deform the surface.

In the subject literature there are few papers describing the use of cryoablation in the treatment of vasomotor rhinitis, which shows that this alternative procedure seems to have been forgotten.

Strome [14] describes cryotherapy as an effective treatment. Improvement of nasal obstruction was observed in 85.7% patients with vasomotor rhinitis. Cryoablation is particularly effective in chronic non-allergic rhinitis with hypertrophy of inferior nasal turbinate.

Jurkiewicz et al. [13] also emphasized the advantages of cryosurgery in treating non-allergic rhinitis.

Rakover and Rosen [15] studied the effects of cryosurgery in treating hypertrophy of inferior nasal turbinates; they observed improvement of nasal obstruction in 62% patients.

Ligezinski et al. [16] stressed the use of cryosurgery in nasal obstruction as the method is effective and significantly improves patient quality of life.

Hartley and Willatt [17] also successfully used cryosurgery in nasal obstruction due to the hypertrophy of inferior nasal the turbinates in adults and stressed that cryosurgery, being safe, may replace more radical surgical methods. Wengraf [18] compared two methods of treatment, diathermy and cryosurgery, and confirmed that the use of cryotherapy in nasal obstruction is a safe method which does not result in complications.

Good effects after cryoablation were also obtained in patients with nasal obstruction in the course of allergic rhinitis, particularly chronic all year round allergic rhinitis.

Zawisza [5] used cryoablation in a patient who had unsuccessfully been treated for nasal obstruction for some years. A year after the procedure the patient was no-longer taking any drugs and was breathing freely through the nose. Three months after cryoablation, Zielinska-Blizniewska et al. [19] observed improvement of nasal obstruction in 63.3% patients with allergic and 76.7% with non-allergic rhinitis.

CONCLUSION

Cryosurgery is a safe and painless, with no bleeding method recommended for chronic allergic and non-allergic rhinitis; it improves patient quality of life. The procedure may be used in an outpatient clinic and does not require premedication. It is an alternative to other treatments, including pharmacotherapy.

REFERENCES

[1] Bracco, D.: The historic development of cryosurgery. *Clin. Dermatol.* 1990, 1, 1-4.

[2] Freiman, A., Bouganim, N.: History of cryotherapy. *Dermatology in Gene Medicine* 1999: 2980-2987.

[3] Gage, A.: History of Cryosurgery. *Semin. Surg. Oncol.* 1998, 14, 99-109.

[4] Hartley, C., Willatt, D. J.: Cryotherapy in the treatment of nasal obstruction: indications in adults. *J. Laryngol. Otol.* 1995, 109(8), 729-732.

[5] Hicks, J. N.: Office treatment by cryotherapy for severe posterior nasal epistaxis. *Laryngoscope* 1983, 93, 876-879.

[6] Hill, C. L.: Preliminary report of cryosurgery in otolaryngology. *Laryngoscope* 1966, 76, 109-111.

[7] Jurkiewicz, D., Zielnik-Jurkiewicz, B.: Non-allergic rhinitis. *Therapy* 2004, 4, 31-34.

[8] Krecicki, T.: *The use of cryosurgery in otolaryngology (in) Cryotherapy in medicine.* Gabrys, M. S., Popiela, A., Urban and Partner, Wroclaw, 2003, 80-92.

[9] Ligezinski, A., Jurkiewicz, D., Hermanowski, M.: Experiences in the treatment of chronic rhinitis by cryoapllication AK-1. *Military Doctor*, 1993, 3, 240-245.

[10] Miszka, K.: Cryotherapy in treatment diseases of otolaryngology. *Nowa Medycyna* 1966, 3, 49-51.

[11] Moszynski, B., Miszka, K.: *Cryotherapy in otorynolaryngology*. PZWL Warsaw 1984.

[12] Popiela, A., Chorowski, M.: *Cryotherapy and cryosurgery – history (in) Cryotherapy in medicine*. Gabrys, M. S., Popiela, A., Urban and Partner, Wroclaw, 2003, 1-4.

[13] Rabin, Y., Coleman, R., Mordohovich, D., Ber, R., Shitzer, A.: A new cryosurgical device for controlled freezing. *Cryobiology*, 1996 Feb., 33 (1): 93-105.

[14] Rakover, Y., Rosen, G.: A comparison of partial inferior turbinectomy and cryosurgery for hypertrophic inferior turbinates. *Journal of Laryngology and Otology*, v. 110, n. 8 (1996): 732-735.

[15] Strome, M.: A long-term assessment of cryotherapy for treating vasomotor intability. *Ear Nose Throat J*. 1990, 69(12), 839-842.

[16] Wengraf, C. L., Gleeson, M. L., Siodlak, M. Z.: The stuffy nose: a comparative study of two common methods of treatment. *Clin. Otolaryng. Allied Sci.*, 1986, 11(2), 61-68.

[17] Zakrzewska, J. M.: Cryotherapy for trigeminal neuralgia: a 10 year audit. *Br. Journal Oral Maxillofac. Surg.*, 1991 Feb., v. 1: 29(1): 1-4.

[18] Zawisza, E.: Cryosurgery in rhinoallergology. *Allergy* 2006, 3, 24-26.

[19] Zielinska-Blizniewska, H., Repetowski, M., Milonski, J., Olszewski, J.: Comparative assessment of cryosurgical treatment results in allergic and non-allergic rhinitis. *Otolaryng. Pol.* 2011, 65(4), 276-280.

In: Cryosurgery and Colposcopy
Editor: Lillian Watson

ISBN: 978-1-63484-507-6
© 2016 Nova Science Publishers, Inc.

Chapter 2

CRYOSURGERY IN RENAL TUMORS

Amr Soliman Moustafa, MD, MSc,
and Ahmed Kamel Abdel-Aal, MD, MSc, PhD*
Department of Radiology, University of Alabama at Birmingham
Birmingham, Alabama, US

ABSTRACT

The percentages of incidentally discovered renal cell carcinoma (RCC) has increased recently due to the routine use of cross-sectional imaging in the diagnosis and follow up of different diseases. More than 50% of incidentally discovered RCCs are diagnosed in patients with advanced age, which is an age group associated with multiple co-morbidities. Luckily, most RCCs are incidentally discovered at a very early stage (Stage 1A). The combination of early stage disease and multiple co-morbidities favored nephron sparing minimal invasive surgeries, such as ablation techniques. Cryosurgery plays an important role in the management of these patients and became one of the standard of care options for management of stage 1A RCC. When performed either percutaneously or laparoscopically, cryosurgery is considered the most frequently used ablative technique in management of RCC. Furthermore, cryosurgery has been well reported in the management of other non-RCC renal tumors.

In this chapter, we aim to address all clinical aspects of cryosurgery including indications, selection criteria, contraindications, technical

---

* Email: akamel@uabmc.edu, 619 19th Street South, Birmingham, AL 35249.

procedure considerations, complications, and post treatment follow up. We will summarize the current status of cryosurgery in the treatment guidelines along with the technical success and clinical outcomes of this technique, and compare it to other ablative techniques including the most recent ones such as irreversible electroporation (IRE), and high-intensity focused ultrasound (HIFU). Furthermore, we will discuss the future perspectives of cryosurgery in management of small renal tumors.

1. INTRODUCTION

In the era of advancement in medical imaging, diagnosis and follow up of diseases became more and more dependent on cross-sectional imaging. Recently, 50% of diagnosed RCCs are found to be incidentally detected in asymptomatic patients during unrelated cross sectional imaging [1]. Luckily, most of the incidentally diagnosed RCCs are detected in their early-stage. Small renal masses (SRMs) are defined as any renal lesion measuring less than 3 cm in diameter. The SRMs includes benign renal lesions such as lipid-poor angiomyolipoma and oncocytoma. However, 80% of the SRMs are proven to be RCCs [2].

Three factors are taken into consideration in the management of SRMs: control of malignancy, preservation of renal function, and patients' co-morbidities. Nephron-sparing minimally invasive techniques, such as ablation techniques, play an important role in recent management of SRMs. Since 50% of incidentally discovered RCCs are diagnosed in elderly patients and most of these RCCs are diagnosed at early stage (Stage 1A), ablation techniques became the mainstay in management of these renal masses [3-6].

Many thermal and non-thermal ablation techniques have been used in clinical practice. Cryosurgery, a thermal ablation technique, had been reported to successfully ablate malignant and benign renal masses such as RCCs and angiomyolipoma [7].

Cryoablation can be performed through either percutaneous or laparoscopic approach. Selection of the preferable approach is mainly dependent on tumor location in the kidney, adjacency to a nearby organ, and the general condition of the patient [8]. The mechanism of action of cryosurgery is through rapid cooling of the tissue below -30 to -40°C which result in ice-ball formation. Alternating freezing and thawing cycles are applied that eventually will result in cell death through tissue disruption, cell rupture, and tissue ischemia [9, 10].

The key to successful cryoablation is mainly dependent on precise preoperative tumor mapping and localization through preoperative CT or MRI, precise placement of the cryoprobe, monitoring of the ice-ball through intra-procedural imaging guidance either by CT or US, and repetition of cooling and thawing cycles [8, 11].

2. HISTORICAL BACKGROUND

While using cold in medicine dates back to ancient Egyptian and Greek civilizations, James Arnott was the 1st one to report local use of cryosurgery between 1891-1979 as a palliative management of skin, breast and cervical tumors. He designed his own equipment using a mixture of salt and crushed ice to reduce pain and local hemorrhage [12, 13].

Campbell White was the first to use refrigerants in medical practice at the late 19th century. He used liquid air in treatment of skin carcinoma. Carbon dioxide snow was used in cryosurgery nearly at the same time period by William Pusey as a therapeutic treatment of skin navi and other benign dermal conditions. The first use of cryosurgery in deeply seated lesions was associated with the technological development of liquid nitrogen as a refrigerant. Irving Cooper was the first one to perform cryosurgical ablation of the thalamus in patient with Parkinson's disease and other non-operable brain tumors by a specially designed liquid nitrogen probe at the early twenty's century [12, 13].

Lutzeyer and Lymberopoulos [14] performed the first experimental cryoablation study in management of renal malignancy in 1971.

Uchida et al. [15] performed the first percutaneous cryosurgery using a liquid-nitrogen based system in a canine model in 1995. With the advances in technology, the introduction of argon-based cryosurgery and downsizing of the cryoprobe size, cryosurgical ablation of renal tumors became the mainstay in the management of renal malignancy. Nowadays, liquid argon and liquid nitrogen are the most commonly used cryogens [8].

Lately, cryosurgery was introduced as a treatment modality in the management of AML was initiated by Delworth et al. [17], who used a cryoprobe through open surgical incision to ablate a large AML in a patient with solitary kidney.

Byrad et al. [18] published the first case series of cryoablation of AML through laparoscopic approach.

Percutaneous cryoablation of AML was recently reported by Johnson and his colleagues [19] in a case series of patients with solitary kidney.

3. PRINCIPLES OF CRYOSURGERY

The desired cryosurgery cell death can be achieved by performing alternating freezing and thawing cycles. Recent cryosurgery equipment is based on Joule-Thomson effect which is based on cooling of high-pressure gas when it travels into a low-pressure region through a pinhole valve. Most gasses obey this rule as nitrogen and argon, which can reach -196°C and -185°C respectively. Inversely, helium warms as an exception of this rule; therefore, it is used to induce heating during thawing phase [20].

The mechanism of cell death by cryosurgery is classified into acute and chronic events or in other words, direct and delayed vascular effect. Immediate, direct tissue injury is achieved through extracellular ice crystals formation as a result of deep freezing. The extracellular ice crystals formation increase the extracellular osmotic pressure and result in movement of the intracellular contents into the extracellular space which eventually will result in intracellular dehydration, as well as, PH and intracellular composition changes. Intracellular ice crystals formation start to take place after these sequences as a result of breakage of the cell membranes lipid bilayer, which initially prevented the formation of intracellular ice formation [8, 21, 22].

The applied shearing movement of the intracellular ice crystal augmented by cell dehydration perform a direct damage effect to intracellular components and cell membrane which results in cell death. Upon thawing, a process of recrystallization takes place, in which intracellular ice crystals conglomerate together performing a pressure effect that can lead to cell membrane rupture. Melting of extracellular ice crystals creates extracellular hypotonicity which is another mechanism of cell rupture through shifting of extracellular fluids into potentially damaged cells, increasing intracellular pressure and eventually resulting in cell rupture [21, 22].

Delayed vascular injury starts with vasoconstriction in response to freezing cycle which can lead to complete microvascular blood stagnation. Upon thawing, a sequel of vasodilatation, increase permeability, edema, endothelial injury, platelet aggregation and microthrombus formation take place which result in tissue ischemia and cell death [21].

Histological studies of the cryogenic lesions revealed central zone of coagulative necrosis around the cryoprobe surrounded by peripheral zone of partial cell death. In the peripheral zone, a mixture of dead, living and apoptotic cells are seen mixed together. Apoptotic cells are seen when cryogenic cell injury is not strong enough to induce direct cell death but instead, cells linger for a time then starts apoptosis mechanism [23].

Therefore, an ablation safety margin of 1 cm is recommended to ensure complete ablation of the targeted lesion.

4. TECHNIQUE

A. Patient Selection and Pre-Ablation Considerations

The American urological association guidelines recommended cryosurgery as a curative management for small renal masses which is classified as Stage 1A disease. Small renal masses by definition are any renal mass ≤ 3 cm in diameter without extension beyond Gerota's fascia, nodal involvement, or distant metastases. However, with the new cryoprobe technological advancement and multiple cryoprobes technique a curative management became achievable to lesions smaller than 4 cm in diameter. The ideal lesion for cryosurgery would be non-centrally located lesion away from renal sinus, to avoid heat sinking effect from any central vessel [24].

Generally, patients with stage 1A renal tumor are candidates for cryosurgery. However, cryosurgery can be the only surrogate for elderly patients or patients with multiple comorbidities, which make them ineligible for radical or partial nephrectomy.

Other indications include patients with SRMs with solitary or transplanted kidney. Cryosurgery is extremely beneficial in the preservation of renal function in patients with multiple bilateral renal tumors as seen in hereditary conditions such as tuberous sclerosis and Von Hippel-Lindau syndrome.

Relative contraindications of cryoablation include young age, renal sinus tumors, cystic tumors of the kidney, and tumors larger than 4 cm. Critical illness as in sepsis, and intractable coagulation disorder are the two absolute contraindication for cryosurgery [25].

Interdisciplinary team of interventional radiologists and urologists usually evaluate candidates for cryosurgery. Pre-procedure imaging and laboratory investigation are obtained including complete blood picture, international normalized ratio (INR), partial thrombin time (PT), and partial thromboplastin time (PTT).

All anticoagulant and antiplatelet medications should be discontinued for a time sufficient to normalize the coagulation measures. Fresh frozen plasma and platelets can be administrated to patients who show abnormal bleeding profile [26].

B. Probes and Machines

The first generation of cryosurgery machines emerged during the 1960s using liquid nitrogen as a cryogenic agent. In 1990s the second generation of cryosurgery machines was introduced with 3-mm probes using liquid nitrogen. The introduction of argon and helium gasses in cryosurgery led to the 3rd generation of cryosurgery machines which were developed at the early 2000s. A 17- gauge (1.5 mm) probes has emerged with the 3rd generation cryosurgery machines. Different ice-ball shapes can be achieved using different types of cryoprobes depending on the shape of the targeted tumor. Moreover, downsizing of cryoprobes facilitated the use of multiple probes and therefore facilitated ablation of lesions up to 4 cm in its longest dimension [27].

C. Procedure

Preoperative Imaging

Precise tumor mapping, including accurate identification of the anatomical location and relations are quite fundamental to achieve a curative cryoablation of a renal mass. Preoperative imaging is usually obtained including pelvi-abdmonial CT and MRI. Cryoablation are routinely performed through two approaches; laparoscopic and percutaneous approaches.

Laparoscopic Approach

Cryosurgery was performed only through open surgical or laparoscopic approach until the emergence of the percutaneous approach. Nowadays, the laparoscopic approach is only considered in cases where the percutaneous approach is challenging.

A classic transperitoneal or retroperitoneal approach is usually chosen. The protocol of laparoscopic approach includes: free mobilization of kidney within Gerota's fascia, visualization of the renal mass using ultrasound, biopsy of the targeted lesion, positioning of the cryoprobe inside the lesion, and performing the freezing – thawing cycles [25].

The percutaneous approach is now considered as the preferable approach, given the less invasive nature, shorter hospitalization time and the cost-effectiveness of this approach.

However, anterior-located renal masses are preferred to be ablated laparoscopically to avoid injury of adjacent Intra-abdominal organs and blood vessels [28].

Percutaneous Approach

Moderate sedation is the most commonly used anesthesia in percutaneous approach. However, sometimes general anesthesia or deep sedation are required if the patient is on CPAP or on chronic narcotics. Percutaneous biopsies can be obtained before placement of the cryosurgery probe [29]. Currently, the percutaneous approach is considered for posteriorly and laterally located renal masses (Figure 1).

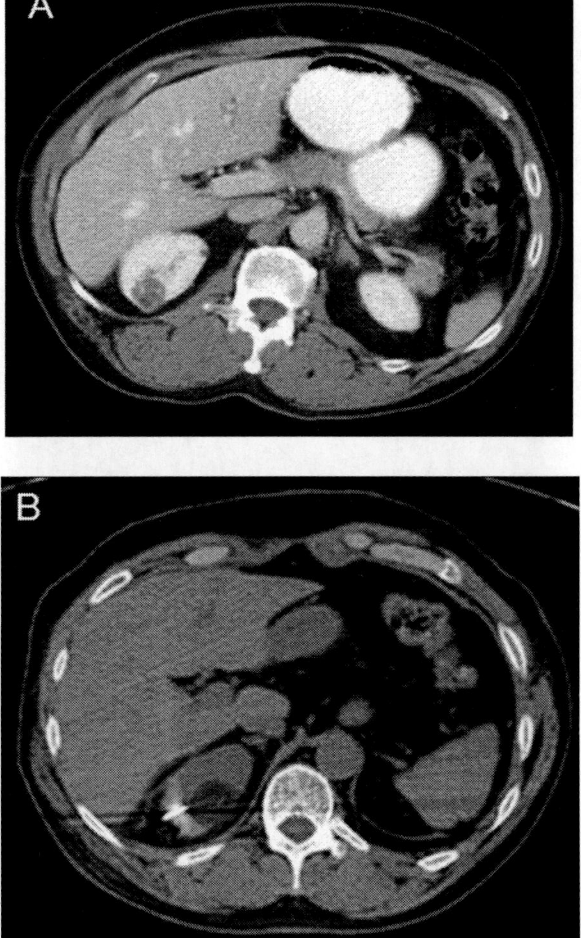

Figure 1. (A) Axial contrast enhanced CT showing a heterogeneously enhancing posterior renal mass. (B) Axial plain CT showing a single percutaneous cryoprobe and evolving ice ball.

With the expertise gained through the wide application of percutaneous cryosurgery, the challenging anteriorly located renal masses became ablateable through percutaneous approach. Mechanical displacement using balloons or hydro-dissection techniques can be performed to separate bowel loops and other intraabdominal organs abutting the targeted renal masses (Figure 2) [29].

Intra-procedural guidance of the cryoprobe and monitoring of the ice-ball formation using ultrasound (US), computerized tomography (CT) or magnetic resonance imaging (MRI) is usually performed.

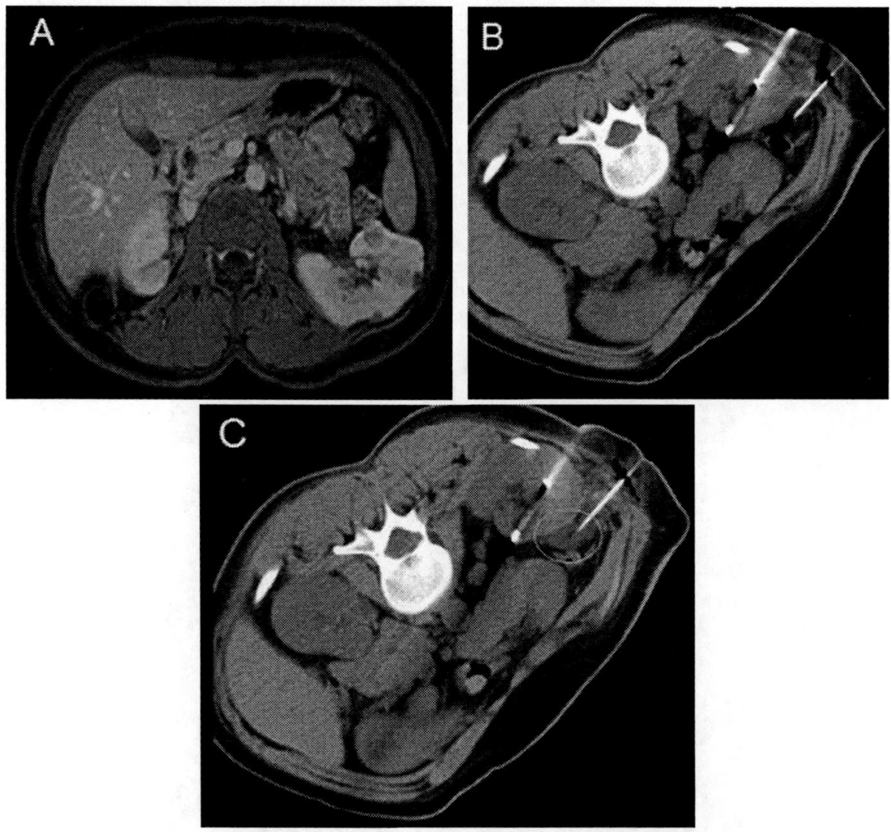

Figure 2. (A) Axial T2 MR image showing close proximity of a bowel loop to an anteriorly located renal mass. (B, C) Hydro-dissection was performed under CT guidance using 40 ml normal saline injected through a 22-G spinal needle achieving an adequate plane of separation between the renal mass and the bowel loop. Note an indwelling cryoprobe.

Ultrasound has the advantage of real-time monitoring of the forming ice-ball in addition to absence of exposure to ionizing radiation. However, ultrasound monitoring can be compromised by several factors including; obese patients, lesions located adjacent to bowel loops or beam attenuation due to the ice-ball formation. Although MRI is the best imaging modality in terms of tissue characterization, cryosurgery using MRI-guidance is rarely performed as there is no wide availability of MRI-compatible cryoprobes [28].

Technical Considerations

The universal protocol of cryoablation consists of 10 to 15 minutes freeze, 8 to 10 minutes thawing phase and then 10 to 15 minutes refreezing. The lethal temperature during the freezing cycle is considered to range from -20 to -40°C. The outer margin of the visible ice-ball contains a non-lethal zone formed at a temperature higher than the lethal range, which does not guarantee total cell death. The extent of this non-lethal zone is measured to be around 5 mm in thickness. Hence, the current recommendation of the ablation zone is to include 5-10 mm beyond the edge of the targeted tumor (Figure 3) [21, 23].

A single or multiple cryoprobes can be used depending on the size and shape of the lesion. In multiple cryoprobes technique, cryoprobes are placed 1.5 cm apart from each other. Three cryoprobes are used to ablate up to 2 cm tumor, while 5 cryoprobes are used to ablate tumors up to 3 cm in size [30].

While rapid cooling during the freezing cycle is an important factor to produce intracellular ice formation resulting in cell death, slow thawing is considered a more important factor in cell necrosis through the re-crystallization process. The repetition of the freezing-thawing cycles is believed to be responsible for 80% of the necrosis of the previously frozen tissue during the initial freezing cycle [21, 23].

Care must be taken with ablation of centrally located renal masses close to the renal sinus to avoid injury of the ureter. Careful monitoring of the ice-ball formation with the possibility of mechanical displacement of the ice-ball by cryoprobe retraction should be performed.

Displacement of the ureter can also be achieved by hydrodissection, CO_2 injection, or even through using a balloon catheter. Other protective measures such as warm pyeloperfusion, in which renal collecting system are irrigated with warm normal saline, can be performed to reduce the probability of ureteric stricture or stenosis following cryosurgery of centrally located renal masses. Moreover, an internal double-J ureteric stents can be placed preoperatively to protect the ureter during ablation and allow ureteral healing in case of cryoinjury [30, 31].

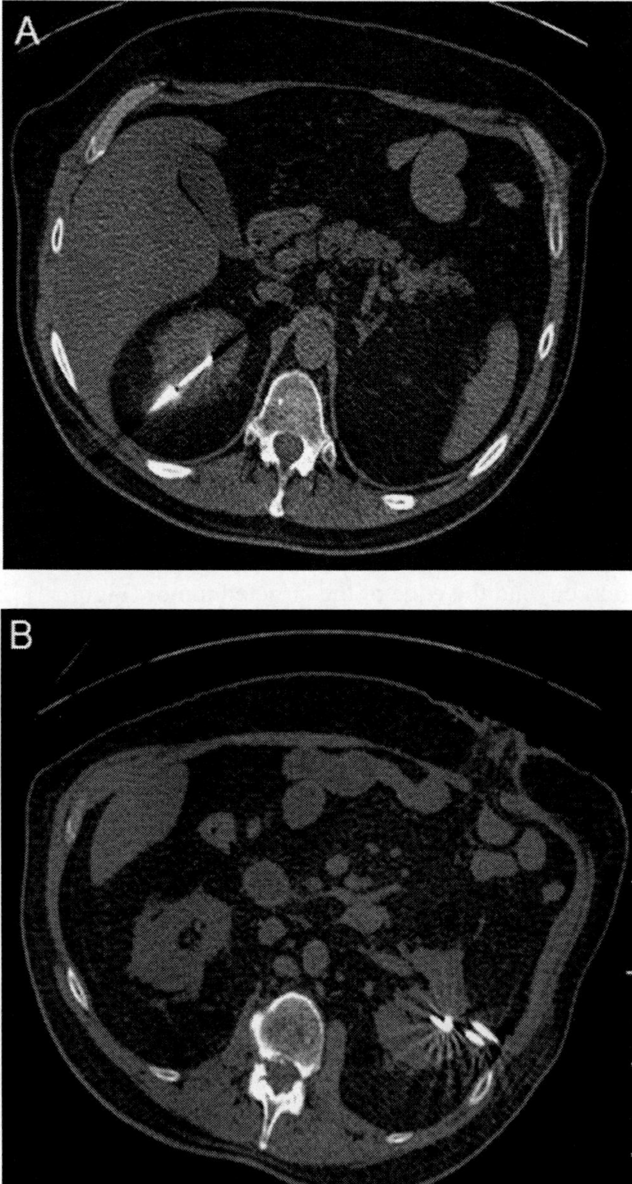

Figure 3. (A, B) Intraprocedural CT showing percutaneous cryoprobes (one on the right and two on the left) at the sites of the renal masses. Note the position of the cryoprobes slightly beyond the margin of the tumor to achieve an ice ball of at least 5-10 mm beyond the tumor margin.

Post Treatment Imaging and Follow Up

There is no algorithm for post-cryosurgery follow-up, however, traditionally imaging are obtained every 3-month interval up to 18 months and then annually for 5 years or until complete disappearance of the ablated lesion.

Contrast-enhanced MRI or CT is the most commonly used in the imaging follow up of these patients [32]. Initially, during short-term follow-up after ablation, the size of the lesion is expected to be seen larger in comparison to pre-ablation size.

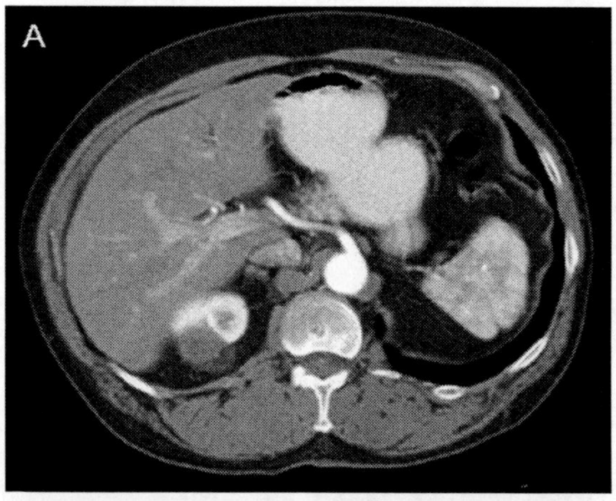
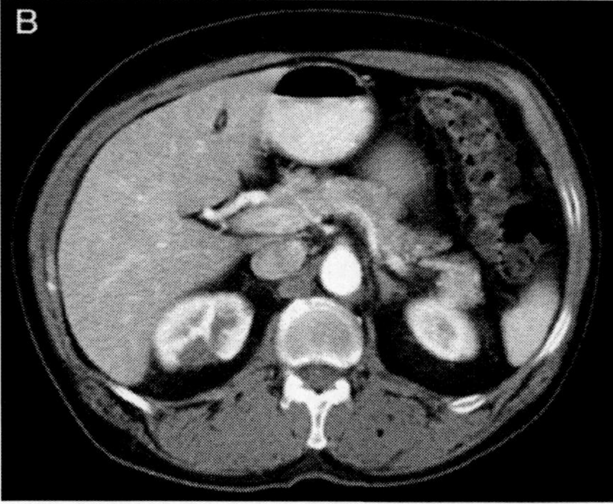

Figure 4. (A) Axial post ablation contrast enhanced CT showing no residual enhancement. There is stranding of the perinephric fat. (B) Axial contrast enhanced CT 6 months later showing decreased size of the ablation zone with no residual enhancement.

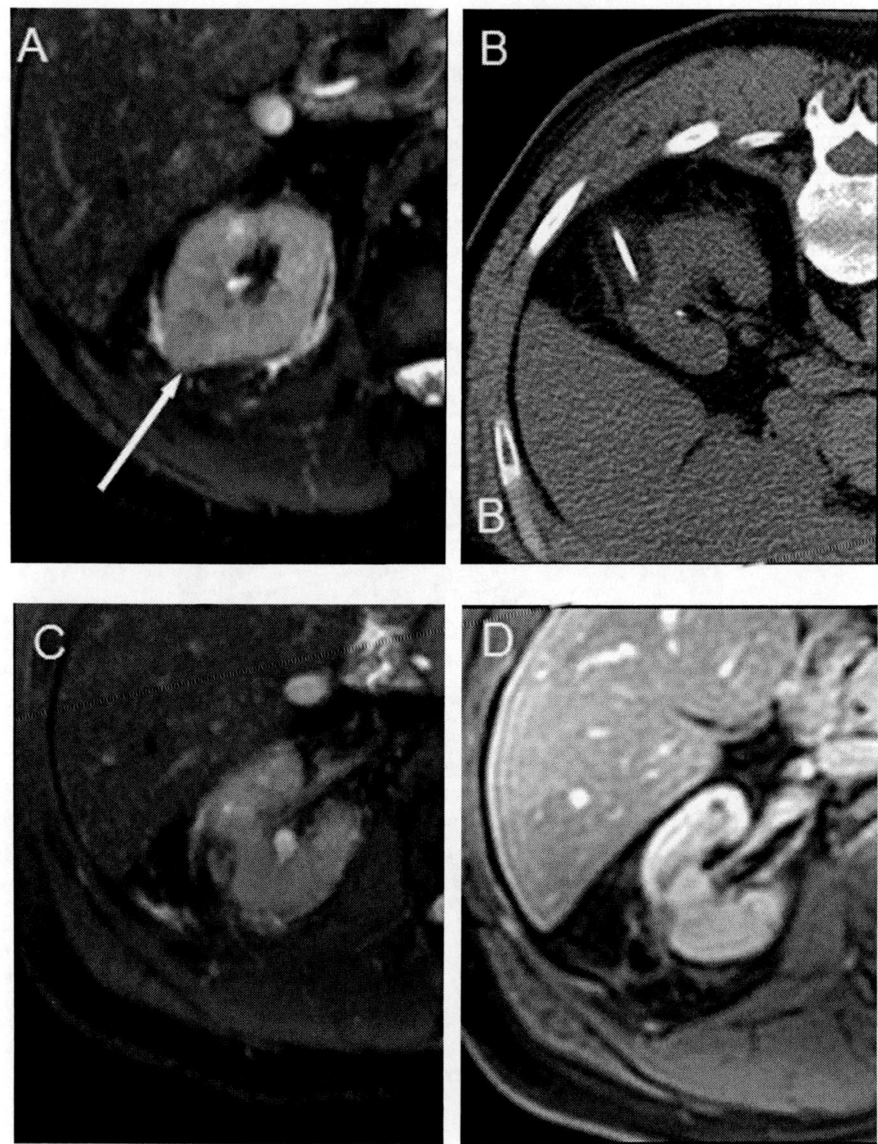

Figure 5. (A) Axial T2 MR image showing a hypointense posterior interpolar renal mass (arrow). (B) Intraprocedural plain CT image showing a single percutaneous cryoprobe and evolving ice ball. (C) Axial T2 MR image 5 months later showing decrease in the size of the ablation zone. (D) Post contrast T1 MR image showing no enhancement. There are surrounding post ablation changes in the perinephric fat.

The extent of the ice-ball beyond the ablated tumor margin and the postoperative fibrosis sequel are the reason behind tumor size increase. Decrease in tumor size and the absence of residual enhancement indicate a favorable post-ablative response. Regression in tumor size can take up to many years till complete disappearance is accomplished (Figure 4 and 5).

Post-operative failure of progressive decrease in tumor size or persistence of tumor enhancement indicate treatment failure and necessitates further intervention (Figure 6) [32].

Complications

Cryosurgery of renal masses is associated with low rate of complications. The most commonly reported complications are pain and paresthesia at the cryoprobe insertion site. Subcapsular and perinephric hemorrhage are also considered common complications of renal cryosurgery (Figure 7). However, it is mostly self-limited, if the coagulation profile is within an acceptable range. Centrally located tumors are associated with increased risk of hematuria, due to its close proximity to the renal sinus [26].

Percutaneous cryoablation of upper pole renal masses is associated with increased risk of pneumothorax.

However, this should not hinder performing the procedure, as in-situ chest tube can be placed if there was a clinical indication. Cryoablation of upper pole renal masses are also associated with increased risk of cardiovascular complications which might be explained by the over-release of catecholamines resulting from adrenal gland stimulation. Adrenal crisis is also a reported complication when cryoablation is performed for tumors that are located near the adrenal glands [33].

Cryoablation of non-targeted lesion is mostly seen with ureters and bowel loops. Careful approach can usually minimize these inadvertent complications. The risk of urinary tract infection is extremely low [31].

5. OUTCOMES

The current guidelines set partial nephrectomy as the gold standard for management of Stage 1A renal tumors.

However, the results of recent long-term studies and meta-analyses have demonstrated very comparable results to renal cryoablation in selected patient population [34, 35].

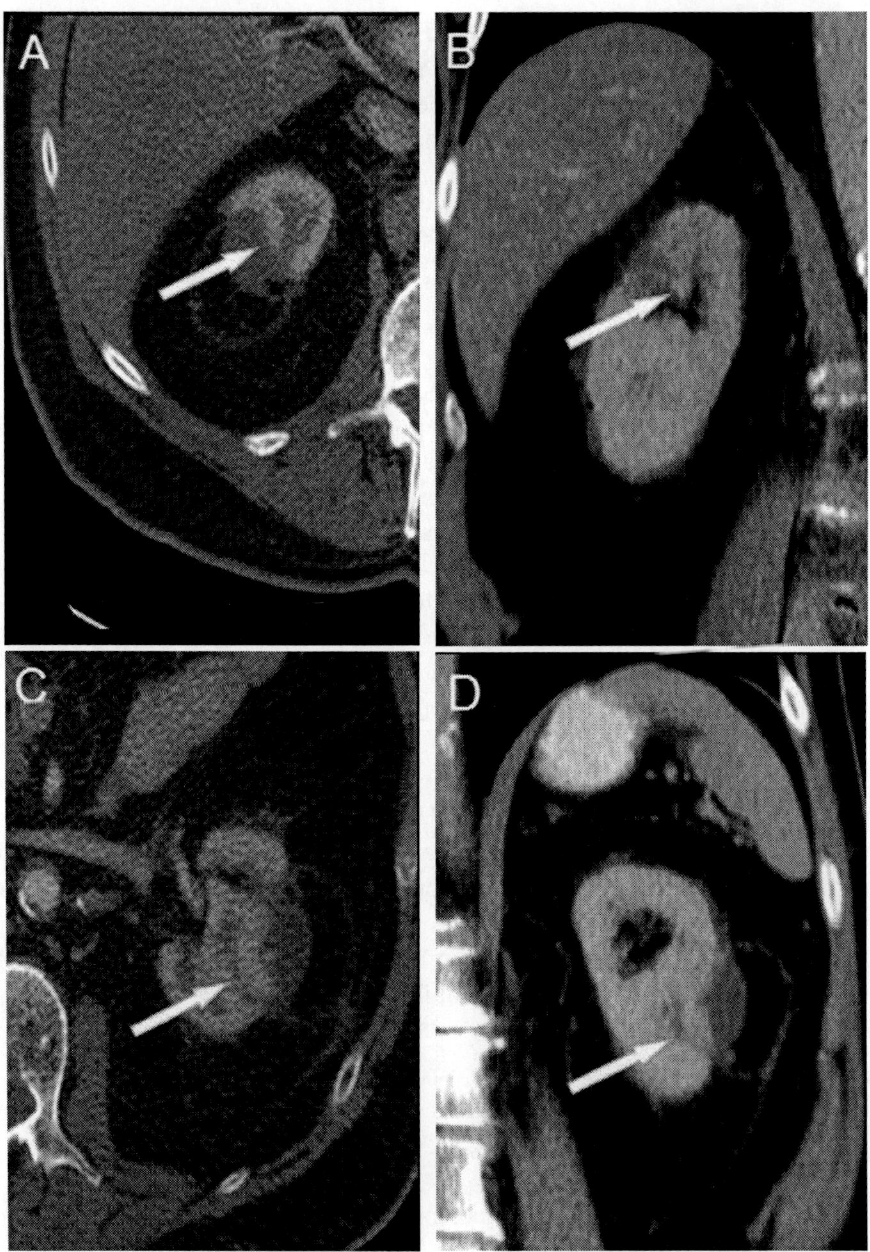

Figure 6. Axial (A) and coronal (B) contrast enhanced CT 3 months following cryoablation of renal cell carcinoma showing nodular central enhancement concerning for residual tumor. Axial (C) and coronal (D) contrast enhanced CT 3 months later showing medial curvilinear enhancement concerning for residual tumor.

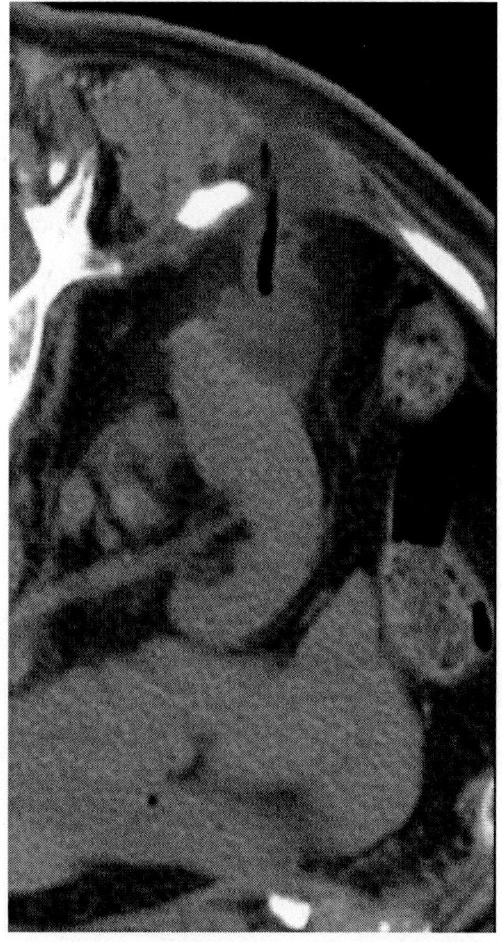

Figure 7. Post ablation non-contrast CT showing cryoprobe track with surrounding small perinephric hematoma and stranding of the perinephric fat.

Oncologic Outcomes

A systematic review ran by Kapoor et al. [36] evaluating cryoablation results in management of SRMs demonstrated a disease-free survival ranging between 84.3% and 100% with mean follow–up of 64 months. Similarly, Klatte and his colleagues [37] published comparable results in their meta-analysis with disease-free survival of more than 90% with a mean follow-up of 29 months.

Treatment failure defined by local tumor recurrence after cryoablation of renal tumors ranged between 4.6% and 5.2% as reported in two meta-analyses [38, 39].

A systematic review demonstrated a higher local tumor recurrence in lesion treated by cryoablation as compared to lesion treated by partial nephrectomy with a relative risk of 7.45. Another systematic review demonstrated similar results with a 4.82 relative risk of local tumor recurrence after cryoablation compared to partial nephrectomy [37].

Although Kunkle and his colleagues demonstrated a higher risk of tumor recurrence in renal lesions treated by cryosurgery, there was not significant difference between both groups regarding the progression to metastatic disease. However, Tang et al. [40] showed a higher local recurrence and a higher distant metastasis with cryosurgery compared to partial nephrectomy.

A significant selection bias is observed in the published literature when comparing the oncologic outcomes of cryosurgery versus partial nephrectomy, since cryosurgery was performed more in elderly patients with poor prognosis and in patients with solitary kidney.

However, the current available data demonstrates similar rates of disease control in terms of disease-specific mortality, disease-free mortality, and overall mortality despite of the higher rates of local tumor recurrence in cases treated with cryosurgery compared to partial nephrectomy [36, 40].

The use of cryosurgery in ablating benign renal masses has not been widely performed. Limited numbers of small case series have been published. These studies demonstrated safety and efficacy of cryosurgery in management of AMLs, more specifically in patients with solitary kidney (Figure 8) [19, 7, 18].

Functional Outcomes

Although the oncologic outcome is the primary outcome in the management of cancer patients, preservation of renal functions is a crucial factor in dealing with renal tumors, especially in patients with solitary kidney, bilateral renal tumors, and patients with chronic renal diseases. Many reports suggested preservation of renal functions after renal cryosurgery at both short and long-term follow-up [41-44].

Comparing functional outcomes after cryosurgery, as a nephron-sparing treatment modality, to the standard partial nephrectomy for stage 1A renal tumors has been published by several authors.

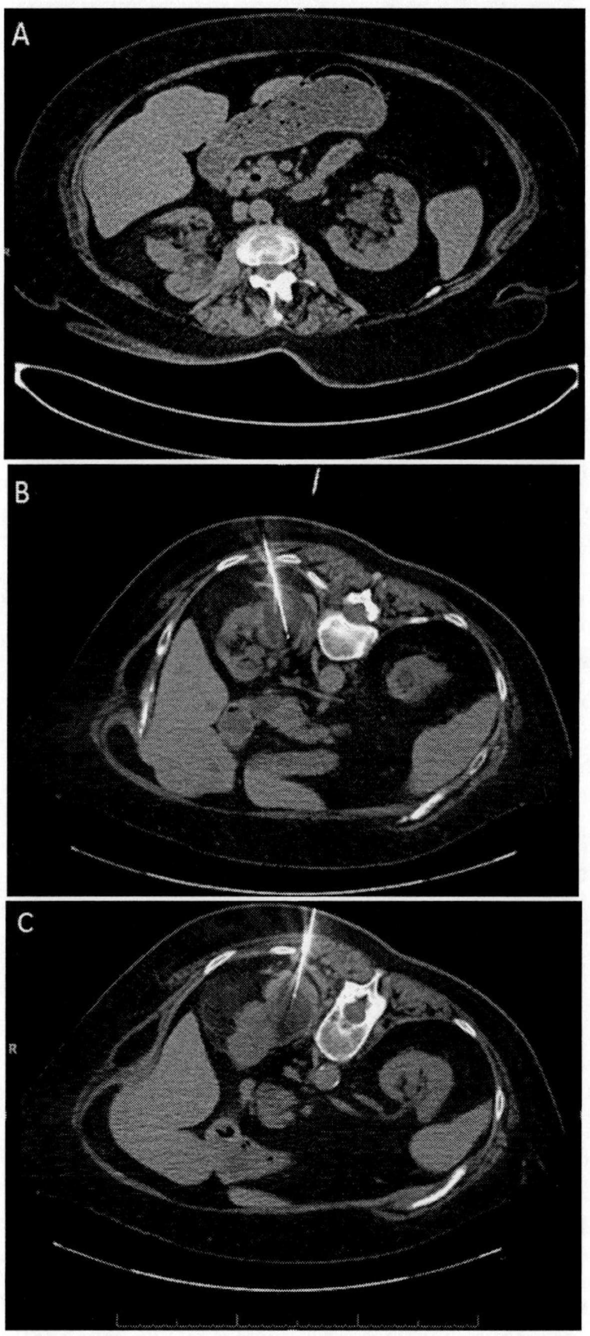

Figure 8. (Continued).

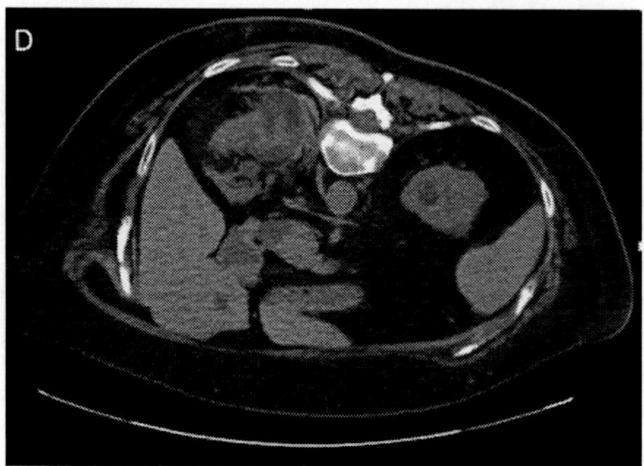

Figure 8. (a) Axial CT image in a patient with multiple bilateral renal angiomyolipomas demonstrating a large, 4.5 cm exophytic angiomyolipoma from the right kidney. (b) and (c) Axial CT images during cryoablation with two cryoprobes positioned in the angiomyolipoma. (d) Axial CT image in the same patient after cryoablation.

Tanagho and his colleagues [45] retrospectively evaluated patients with SRMs and suggested a significantly less decline in glomerular filtration rate GFR in the cryosurgery group (n = 267) compared to the partial nephrectomy group (n = 233). Conversely, Panumatrassame et al. [46] demonstrated no significant difference in the GFR between both groups.

Of note, Panumatrassame et al. suggested a better perioperative outcome with less blood loss, shorter hospital stay, and fewer complications in the cryosurgery group [46]. In a meta-analysis done by Tang et al. [40], data pooling from 9 published trials confirmed these results and demonstrated no significant difference in the postoperative serum Creatinine and GFR between cryosurgery and partial nephrectomy.

Percutaneous and Laparoscopic Cryosurgery Outcomes

Percutaneous cryosurgery became the popular approach given the shorter hospital stay and the significant cost advantages over the laparoscopic approach [47-49].

Although a lower technical success rate and a higher local tumor recurrence rate were observed with percutaneous cryosurgery, there was no significant difference in the survival outcomes. This might be due to the repetition of cryoablation [50, 51].

Long and colleagues concluded that cryoablation provides similar oncologic outcomes regardless of the approach in their published systematic review [52].

Cryosurgery versus Other Ablative Techniques

Different ablative techniques are available for clinical use. Cryosurgery has the advantages of real-time visualization of the "ice-ball" corresponding to the future ablation zone, less post-procedure pain due to its intrinsic anesthetic effects, and the ability to use multiple probes simultaneously.

However, there are many disadvantages inherent to this modality compared to radiofrequency ablation such as; longer procedure time and the inability to cauterize the probe tract resulting in a theoretically increased risk of bleeding.

However, the overall risk of bleeding from cryosurgery of renal tumors is relatively low because of its retroperitoneal location and the tamponade effect of Gerota's fascia [31].

Radiofrequency

Radiofrequency ablation (RF) is a widely used ablative technique in clinical practice. The basic principal of RF is generating heat (Temperature up to 100°C) through passing a high-frequency alternating current through an electrode to induce necrosis of the targeted lesion [31].

The main advantage of RF over cryosurgery is the inherent cautery effect. This can be used to minimize bleeding by cauterization of the ablation tract. The short procedure time (6-20 min) is another advantage, compared to cryoablation (25 minutes) [31, 53].

The main drawback of RF is the "heat sink effect," which results from heat dispersion when RF is applied to a lesion close to a high-flow blood vessel. Such phenomenon limits the application of RF ablation in lesions located close to blood vessels. Another limitation of RF ablation is reported in cystic lesions [31, 53].

Pirasteh and colleagues [54] reported no significant difference between RF and cryosurgery regarding oncologic efficacies. The authors also noted no changes in the baseline renal functions after performing either RF or cryoablation. These data were confirmed by another study performed by Pettus et al. [55].

Microwave

Ablation using microwave has been recently introduced in US. Microwave antennas use electromagnetic waves to produce an electromagnetic field that result in heat production which can reach up to 150°C. The theoretical superiority of microwave over RF is due to the non-necessity of direct physical contact between tissue and the microwave antenna; therefore, a deeper tissue penetration can be achieved. Microwave can replace RF ablation in lesions with potential heat sink effect [31, 56].

Yu and colleagues [57] reported their mid-term results with microwave ablation of RCCs, with a technical effectiveness of 98%, 3-year local tumor progression rate of 7.7%, and cancer-specific survival at 3 years of 97.8%. These data are comparable to cryosurgery and RF. However, another recent study demonstrated disappointing results for renal tumor microwave ablation. The investigators of this study presented tumor recurrence rate of 38% at 18-month follow-up. In addition, a high intraoperative and postoperative complication rate was observed [58].

Guan et al. [59] reported a prospective randomized study comparing microwave ablation to partial nephrectomy. Comparable oncologic results were observed. However, a postoperative deterioration of renal function was noted in the microwave group.

Irreversible Electroporation (IRE)

Irreversible electroporation (IRE) is a non-thermal ablation induced by the application of rapid electrical pulses which results in the creation of microscopic pores are created within the cell membranes. Being a non-thermal ablation technique, it is not susceptible to the "heat sink effect" and has the potential for relative urothelial protection. However, the lack of cauterization of the entry tract increases the possibility of bleeding and tract seeding. In addition, potential cardiac arrhythmia and muscle contractions necessitate intra-procedure electrocardiographic monitoring and neuromuscular blockade [31, 60]. Recent studies suggested the safety of IRE in ablating renal masses. However, many studies are warranted to measure its efficacy and compare it to other established techniques [60].

High-Intensity Focused Ultrasound (HIFU)

The basic principal of this ablative technique is the induction of heat through a high-power, highly focused ultrasound beams targeting a specific point within the body. The ultrasound beams produce heat (50°C) through tissue vibration. The generated heat is sufficient to induce tissue necrosis.

Intra- and extracorporeal HIFU systems are available. While intracorporeal systems are used in open and laparoscopic surgery, the extracorporeal systems are ultrasound or MRI guided. The extracorporeal HIFU system has the advantage of being entirely non-invasive unlike other ablative techniques. Therefore, there is no potential risk of tract hemorrhage or tumor seeding [61]. Many technical limitations hinder the clinical use of extracorporeal HIFU such as respiratory movement, different depth of the targeted lesion, and tissue variability. The application of intracorporeal HIFU could abolish some of these limitations. However, recent publications demonstrated disappointing results with limited percent of complete therapeutic tissue necrosis of the target renal tumor [60-62].

Recent Advances in Cryosurgery

Recent advances in ablation techniques focus on improving precise probe positioning, minimizing treatment-related complications and maximizing the energy delivered to the targeted lesion [8].

Real-time virtual ultrasonography (RVS) (Hitachi Medical Corporation, Tokyo, Japan) is a new software technique to allow better intraprocedural visualization of the target tumor. This technique allows fusion of intraprocedural real-time ultrasonography with preoperative, preloaded CT scan of the same area of the body. The main advantage of this technique is to overcome the decrease in US quality during the cryosurgery procedure [8].

In an attempt to minimize laparoscopic ports and decrease any potential associated morbidity, Single port access renal cryoablation (SPARC) has been recently introduced, in which a multichannel single port is inserted through the umbilicus. Goel and colleagues [63] published their initial data on SPARC which demonstrated encouraging results with no complications.

CONCLUSION

Recent publications demonstrated an expanding trend in the use of thermal and non-thermal ablative techniques for the management of renal masses. Cryoablation and RF ablation are the most clinically implemented and the most studied modalities. Data suggest that cryosurgery has a comparable oncologic result to the standard partial nephrectomy when used for the treatment of small renal masses.

Cryosurgery oncologic outcomes, functional outcomes and complications were the same regardless of the approach. While there is no statistical difference between cryosurgery and RF ablation regarding ablation of renal masses, the use of either modality is largely dependent on physician preference and personal experience, in addition to the availability within the institution. Finally, the newly introduced ablative techniques such as Microwave, IRE and HIFU have some theoretical advantages over the more studied Cryosurgery and RF. However, the outcomes from the available studies are not encouraging which warrants future prospective studies with long-term outcomes to evaluate their efficacy.

REFERENCES

[1] Jayson, M., Sanders, H. Increased incidence of serendipitously discovered renal cell carcinoma. *Urology* 1998;51(2):203-205.

[2] Homma, Y., Kawabe, K., Kitamura, T., Nishimura, Y., Shinohara, M., Kondo, Y. et al. Increased incidental detection and reduced mortality in renal cancer - recent retrospective analysis at eight institutions. *Int. J. Urol.* 1995;2(2):77-80.

[3] El Dib, R., Touma, N. J., Kapoor, A. Cryoablation vs radiofrequency ablation for the treatment of renal cell carcinoma: a meta-analysis of case series studies. *BJU Int.* 2012;110(4):510-516.

[4] Tracy, C. R., Raman, J. D., Donnally, C., Trimmer, C. K., Cadeddu, J. A. Durable oncologic outcomes after radiofrequency ablation: experience from treating 243 small renal masses over 7.5 years. *Cancer* 2010;116:3135-3142.

[5] Bandi, G., Hedican, S. P., Nakada, S. Y. Current practice patterns in the use of ablation technology for the management of small renal masses at academic centers in the United States. *Urology* 2008;71(1):113-117.

[6] Hinshaw, J. L., Shadid, A. M., Nakada, S. Y., Hedican, S. P., Winter, T. C. III, Lee, F. T. Jr. Comparison of percutaneous and laparoscopic cryoablation for the treatment of solid renal masses. *AJR Am. J. Roentgenol.* 2008;191(4):1159-1168.

[7] Sivalingam, S., Nakada, S. Y. Contemporary minimally invasive treatment options for renal angiomyolipomas. *Curr. Urol. Rep.* 2013;14 (2):147-53.

[8] Autorino, R. 1., Kaouk, J. H. Cryoablation for small renal tumors: current status and future perspectives. *Urol. Oncol.* 2012 (4 Suppl.):S20-27.

[9] Hoffmann, N. E., Bischof, J. C. The cryobiology of cryosurgical injury. *Urology* 2002;60:40-49.

[10] Woolley, M. L., Schulsinger, D. A., Durand, D. B. et al. Effect of freezing parameters (freeze cycle and thaw process) on tissue destruction following renal cryoablation. *J. Endourol.* 2002;16:519-522.

[11] Theodorescu, D. Cancer cryotherapy: evolution and biology. *Rev. Urol.* 2004;6(Suppl. 4):S9-S19.

[12] Andrew, A. G. History of Cryosurgery. *Seminars in Surgical Oncology* 1998; 14:99-109.

[13] Cooper, S. M., Dawber, R. P. The history of cryosurgery. *J. R. Soc. Med.* 2001;94(4):196-201.

[14] Lutzeyer, W., Lymberopoulos, S. The cryoscalpel for renal surgery: an experimental study. *Invest. Urol.* 1971;8(4):462-77.

[15] Uchida, M., Imaide, Y., Sugimoto, K., Uehara, H., Watanabe, H. Percutaneous cryosurgery for renal tumours. *Br. J. Urol.* 1995;75:132-136.

[16] Uzzo, R. G., Novick, A. C. Nephron-sparing surgery for renal tumors: Indications, techniques and outcomes. *J. Urol.* 2001;166:6-18.

[17] Delworth, M. G., Pisters, L. L., Fornage, B. D., von Eschenbach, A. C. Cryotherapy for renal cell carcinoma and angiomyolipoma. *J. Urol.* 1996;155(1):252-254.

[18] Byrd, G. F., Lawatsch, E. J., Mesrobian, H. G., Begun, F., Langenstroer, P. Laparoscopic cryoablation of renal angiomyolipoma. *J. Urol.* 2006; 176(4 Pt 1):1512-1516.

[19] Johnson, S. C., Graham, S., D'Agostino, H., Elmajian, D. A., Shingleton, W. B. Percutaneous renal cryoablation of angiomyolipomas in patients with solitary kidneys. *Urology.* 2009;74(6):1246-1249.

[20] Williams, S. K., de la Rosette, J., Landman, J., Keeley, F. X. Cryoablation of small renal tumors. *European Association of Urology* 2007;5:206-218.

[21] Gage, A. A., Baust, J. Mechanisms of tissue injury in cryosurgery. *Cryobiology.* 1998;37(3):171-186.

[22] Ahmed, M., Brace, C. L., Lee, F. T. Jr, Goldberg, S. N. Principles of and advances in percutaneous ablation. *Radiology* 2011;258(2):351-369.

[23] Baust, J. G., Gage, A. A. The molecular basis of cryosurgery. *BJU Int.* 2005;95(9):1187-1191.

[24] Zargar, H., Atwell, T. D., Cadeddu, J. A., de la Rosette, J. J., Janetschek, G., Kaouk, J. H. et al. Cryoablation for Small Renal Masses: Selection Criteria, Complications, and Functional and OncologicResults. *Eur. Urol.* 2015. pii: S0302-2838(15)00246-8. doi: 10.1016/j.eururo.2015.03.027.

[25] Schiffman, M., Moshfegh, A., Talenfeld, A., Del Pizzo, J. J. Laparoscopic renal cryoablation. *Semin. Intervent. Radiol.* 2014;31(1): 64-69.

[26] Kurup, A. N. Percutaneous ablation for small renal masses-complications. *Semin. Intervent. Radiol.* 2014 (1):42-9.

[27] Kapoor, A., Wang, Y., Dishan, B., Pautler, S. E. Update on cryoablation for treatment of small renal mass: oncologic control, renal function preservation, and rate of complications. *Curr. Urol. Rep.* 2014;15(4): 396.

[28] Long, C. J., Canter, D. J., Smaldone, M. C., Li, T., Simhan, J., Rozenfeld, B. et al. Role of tumor location in selecting patients for percutaneous versus surgical cryoablation of renalmasses. *Can. J. Urol.* 2012;19(5):6417-6422.

[29] Venkatesan, A. M., Wood, B. J., Gervais, D. A. Percutaneous ablation in the kidney. *Radiology.* 2011;261(2):375-3791.

[30] Georgiades, C., Rodriguez, R. Renal tumor ablation. *Tech. Vasc. Interv. Radiol.* 2013;16(4):230-238.

[31] Webb, H., Lubner, M. G., Hinshaw, J. L. Thermal ablation. *Semin. Roentgenol.* 2011;46(2):133-141.

[32] Kawamoto, S., Solomon, S. B., Bluemke, D. A., Fishman, E. K. Computed tomography and magnetic resonance imaging appearance of renal neoplasms after radiofrequency ablation and cryoablation. *Semin. Ultrasound CT MR.* 2009;30(2):67-77.

[33] Mues, A. C., Landman, J. Image-guided percutaneous ablation of renal tumors: outcomes, technique, and application in urologicpractice. *Curr. Urol. Rep.* 2010;11(1):8-14.

[34] Rioja, J., Tzortzis, V., Mamoulakis, C., Laguna, M. P. Cryotherapy for renal tumors: current status and contemporary developments. *Actas Urol. Esp.* 2010;34(4):309-317.

[35] Khiatani, V., Dixon, R. G. Renal ablation update. *Semin. Intervent. Radiol.* 2014;31(2):157-166.

[36] Kapoor, A., Touma, N. J., Dib, R. E. Review of the efficacy and safety of cryoablation for the treatment of small renal masses. *Can. Urol. Assoc. J.* 2013;7(1):E38-44.

[37] Klatte, T., Grubmüller, B., Waldert, M., Weibl, P., Remzi, M. Laparoscopic cryoablation versus partial nephrectomy for the treatment of small renal masses: systematic review and cumulative analysis of observational studies. *Eur. Urol.* 2011;60(3):435-443.

[38] Kunkle, D. A., Engleston, B. L., Uzzo, R. G. Excise, ablate or observe: The small renal mass dilemma-A meta-analysis and review. *J. Urol.* 2007;179:1227-34.

[39] Kunkle, D. A., Uzzo, R. G. Cryoablation or radiofrequency ablation of the small renal mass. A meta-analysis. *Cancer.* 2008;113:2671-2680.

[40] Tang, K., Yao, W., Li, H., Guo, X., Guan, W., Ma, X. et al. Laparoscopic renal cryoablation versus laparoscopic partial nephrectomy for the treatment of small renalmasses: a systematic review and meta-analysis of comparative studies. *J. Laparoendosc. Adv. Surg. Tech. A.* 2014;24(6):403-410.

[41] Tsivian, M. M., Caso, J., Kimura, M., Polascik, T. J. Renal function outcomes after laparoscopic renal cryoablation. *J. Endourol.* 2011;25(8): 1287-1291.

[42] Tanagho, Y. S., Roytman, T. M., Bhayani, S. B., Kim, E. H., Benway, B. M., Gardner, M. W., Figenshau, R. S. Laparoscopic cryoablation of renal masses: single-center long-termexperience. *Urology* 2012;80(2): 307-314.

[43] Gill, I. S., Remer, E. M., Hasan, W. A., Strzempkowski, B., Spaliviero, M., Steinberg, A. P. et al. Renal cryoablation: outcomes at 3 years. *J. Urol.* 2005;173:1903-1907.

[44] Bourne, A. E., Kramer, B. A., Steiner, H. L., Schwartz, B. F. Renal insufficiency is not a contraindication for cryoablation of small renal masses. *J. Endourol.* 2009;23(7):1195-1198.

[45] Tanagho, Y. S., Bhayani, S. B., Kim, E. H., Figenshau, R. S. Renal cryoablation versus robot-assisted partial nephrectomy: Washington University long-term experience. *J. Endourol.* 2013;27:1477-1486.

[46] Panumatrassamee, K., Kaouk, J. H., Autorino, R. et al. Cryoablation versus minimally invasive partial nephrectomy for small renal masses in the solitary kidney: impact of approach on functional outcomes. *J. Urol.* 2013;189(3):818-822.

[47] Finley, D. S., Beck, S., Box, G. et al. Percutaneous and laparoscopic cryoablation of small renal masses. *J. Urol.* 2008;180:492-498.

[48] Bandi, G., Hedican, S., Moon, T., Lee, F. T., Nakada, S. Y. Comparison of postoperative pain, convalescence, and patient satisfaction after laparoscopic and percutaneous ablation of small renal masses. *J. Endourol.* 2008;22(5):963-967.

[49] Badwan, K., Maxwell, K., Venkatesh, R., Figenshau, R. S., Brown, D., Chen, C., Bhayani, S. B. Comparison of laparoscopic and percutaneous cryoablation of renal tumors: a cost analysis. *J. Endourol.* 2008;22:1275-1277.

[50] Strom, K. H., Derweesh, I., Stroup, S. P., Malcolm, J. B., L'Esperance, J., Wake, R. W. et al. Second prize: Recurrence rates after percutaneous and laparoscopic renal cryoablation of small renal masses: Does the approach make a difference? *J. Endourol.* 2011;25:371-375.

[51] Malcolm, J. B., Berry, T. T., Williams, M. B., Logan, J. E., Given, R. W., Lance, R. S. et al. Single center experience with percutaneous and laparoscopic cryoablation of small renal masses. *J. Endourol.* 2009;23: 907-911.

[52] Long, C. J., Kutikov, A., Canter, D. J. et al. Percutaneous vs. surgical cryoablation of the small renal mass: Is efficacy compromised? *BJU Int.* 2011;107:1376-80.

[53] Goldberg, S. N., Gazelle, G. S., Mueller, P. R.: Thermal ablation therapy for focal malignancy: a unified approach to underlying principles, techniques, and diagnostic imaging guidance. *AJR Am. J. Roentgenol.* 2000;174:323-331.

[54] Pirasteh, A., Snyder, L., Boncher, N. et al. Cryoablation vs. radiofrequency ablation for small renal masses. *Acad. Radiol.* 2011;18 (1):97-100.

[55] Pettus, J. A., Werle, D. M., Saunders, W., Hemal, A., Kader, A. K., Childs, D., Zagoria, R. J. Percutaneous radiofrequency ablation does not affect glomerular filtration rate. *J. Endourol.* 2010;24(10):1687-1691.

[56] Wright, A. S., Lee, F. T. Jr, Mahvi, D. M. Hepatic microwave ablation with multiple antennae results in synergistically larger zones of coagulation necrosis. *Ann. Surg. Oncol.* 2003;10:275-283.

[57] Yu, J., Liang, P., Yu, X. L. et al. US-guided percutaneous microwave ablation of renal cell carcinoma: intermediate-term results. *Radiology* 2012;263(3):900-908.

[58] Castle, S. M., Salas, N., Leveillee, R. J. Initial experience using microwave ablation therapy for renal tumor treatment: 18-month follow-up. *Urology* 2011;77(4):792-797.

[59] Guan, W., Bai, J., Liu, J. et al. Microwave ablation versus partial nephrectomy for small renal tumors: intermediate-term results. *J. Surg. Oncol.* 2012;106(3):316-321.

[60] Klatte, T., Kroeger, N., Zimmermann, U., Burchardt, M., Belldegrun, A. S., Pantuck, A. J. The contemporary role of ablative treatment approaches in the management of renal cell carcinoma(RCC): focus on radiofrequency ablation (RFA), high-intensity focused ultrasound (HIFU), and cryoablation. *World J. Urol.* 2014;32(3):597-605.

[61] Marberger, M., Schatzl, G., Cranston, D., Kennedy, J. E. Extracorporeal ablation of renal tumours with high-intensity focused ultrasound. *BJU Int.* 2005;95(Suppl. 2):52-55.

[62] Häcker, A., Michel, M. S., Marlinghaus, E., Köhrmann, K. U., Alken, P. Extracorporeally induced ablation of renal tissue by high-intensity focused ultrasound. *BJU Int.* 2006;97(4):779-785.

[63] Goel, R. K., Kaouk, J. H. Single port access renal cryoablation (SPARC): A new approach. *Eur. Urol.* 2008;53:1204-1209.

Section Two: Colposcopy

In: Cryosurgery and Colposcopy
Editor: Lillian Watson

ISBN: 978-1-63484-507-6
© 2016 Nova Science Publishers, Inc.

Chapter 3

THE ROLE OF COLPOSCOPY IN DETECTION AND FOLLOW-UP OF PRE-MALIGNANT CERVICAL LESIONS

Rosekeila Simões Nomelini[*],
*Ana Cristina Macêdo Barcelos, Marcela Moisés Maluf
Sanguinete and Eddie Fernando Candido Murta*
Research Institute of Oncology (IPON);
Discipline of Gynecology and Obstetrics,
Federal University of Triângulo Mineiro (UFTM);
Uberaba, Minas Gerais, Brazil

ABSTRACT

Colposcopy is an important device or method in the diagnosis of cervical lesions and prevention of cervical cancer. Cervical cancer screening programs can be divided into three basic points: screening, management of abnormal cytology and management in post-treatment.

Cervical intraepithelial neoplasia is defined by cellular atypia confined to the epithelium. The screening of these lesions is performed by Pap's smear. This method has good sensitivity and high specificity, but

---

[*] Address for correspondence: Prof. Rosekeila Simões Nomelini, Oncological Research Institute (IPON)/Discipline of Gynecology and Obstetrics, UFTM, Av. Getúlio Guaritá, s/n, Bairro Abadia, 38025-440 Uberaba-MG, Brazil. *e-mail:* rosekeila@terra.com.br.

there is criticism because the rates of false-negative results (10-30%) due to limitations of the procedure. Colposcopy is performed in abnormal cervical cytology. The sensitivity of the test is 85%-96% and specificity around 48%-69%. The specificity and predictive positive value for CIN 2/3 and invasive carcinoma is around 83% and 71.8%, respectively. Colposcopic imaging must evaluate the following parameters: acetowhitening kinetics, vascular pattern and Lugol iodine solution staining (Schiller Test). According to the gradation of the displayed signals, it is estimated the degree of commitment by the injury. Biopsy must be addressed in places where alterations are viewed for definitive diagnosis.

Less than 1% of Pap smear results are diagnosed as atypical glandular cells. These findings are divided by Bethesda System in Atypical Glandular cells of undetermined significance (AGC), adenocarcinoma in situ and invasive adenocarcinoma of uterine cervix. The initial conduct for these patients is very variable and include colposcopy with directed biopsy, endocervical and endometrial curettage. The research of HPV DNA also has an essential role, especially in cases of AGC, which often have significant correlation with clinically important lesions, including invasive adenocarcinoma, identifying those with a higher risk of injury.

In post-treatment, colposcopy is important for monitoring recurrent disease. The main objective of CIN 2/3 excisional treatment is the complete removal of the lesion and transformation zone, leading to a proper interpretation of the margins by the pathologist. The margins status can predict the risk of recurrent disease. The decision of retreatment depends on follow-up with cytology and colposcopy, and some current protocols add HPV biomolecular testing.

Advances in the understanding of cervical carcinogenesis and their relation with the human papillomavirus (HPV) has led to new prevention strategies based on HPV testing. Still, colposcopy remains an important method in the initial evaluation of patients with positive high-risk HPV testing, and realization of cervical biopsy.

INTRODUCTION

Prevention of cervical cancer can be accomplished by abnormal cell detection through Pap smear and subsequent referral for colposcopy and biopsy [1]. Colposcopy is a test that shows the morphology of the cervical mucosa, detecting changes and guiding the biopsy. Moreover, the colposcopic impression has an interobserver variability, and even intraobserver, which is aggravated by the insufficient diffusion of quality assurance [2]. The biopsy of suspected multiple sites by colposcopic examination can be performed to improve the diagnostic accuracy [3].

The aim of this chapter is to address the different colposcopic findings in squamous and glandular cervical lesions, and demonstrate the performance of colposcopy in cervical intraepithelial lesions diagnosis.

SQUAMOUS LESIONS AND HPV

Epidemiology

Cervical cancer is the second most commonly diagnosed cancer and the third leading cause of cancer death in women living in less developed countries. There is a great geographic variation in cancer rates because of the different accesses to screening over the world [4]. According to the latest statistics, USA had 12,042 diagnoses of cervical cancer and 4,074 deaths due to this cancer in 2012 [5].

The decline in the incidence of this disease in the USA is explained by the wide scope and effective form of screening and prevention of this cancer. This reduction is due to the large-scale use of Pap smear. This test has reduced the detection of precancerous lesions significantly [6]. When this examination shows any abnormality, it can be treated and cured in precancerous stage. The cervical cancer prevention protocols envisage Pap smear followed by local biopsies directed by colposcopy, when the image colposcopic shows abnormalities [7].

The causal factor most related to the development of cervical cancer is human papillomavirus (HPV) infection. HPV-16 and HPV-18 subtypes are singled out as the cause of about 70% of cases of cervical cancer. There are over 100 types of HPV, some being related to high risk for carcinogenic evolution. HPV infection can be associated with other genital cancers (vulvar, vaginal, anal, penile cancer), and also non-genital (head and neck cancer). When a woman is infected by HPV, there are two forms of evolution: transient infection and persistent infection. The first is the most common. HPV clearance is due to the action of the immune system against infection. These women don´t have high risk for cervical cancer. These lesions usually manifests as low-grade squamous intraepithelial lesion (LSIL) in Pap smear, and as CIN1/HPV in histology. Persistent infection is less common, but cause greater tissue damage. It manifested through high-grade intraepithelial lesion (HSIL) in cytology and CIN 2 and CIN 3 in histology. They have an increased risk of cervical cancer if they are not identified and treated. In an observational study, 31.3% of women with untreated high-grade lesions progressed to uterine cervical cancer in 30 years of follow-up [6, 7, 8].

The Pap smear has not satisfactory sensitivity rates. For this reason, they are being studied otherways to better screening, diagnosis and early treatment. There is a strong correlation between HPV and cervical lesions, and HPV DNA testing in conjunction with cytology - Pap smears (co-testing) can be utilized. HPV testing is able to identify high-risk HPV types in cervical specimens, and it has a high negative predictive value for CIN diagnosis [9]. The direct referral for colposcopy can also be used in the management of patients with cytological abnormalities [10, 11].

Current guidelines were developed the joint recommendations of the American Cancer Society (ACS), The American Society for Colposcopy and Cervical Pathology (ASCCP) and American Society for Clinical Pathology in 2012, and were accepted and promoted by the American Congress of Obstetricians and Gynecologists (ACOG) in the same year [12]. Current recommendations include:

- Cervical cancer screening shouldn't begin until 21 years old (regardless of age or vaccination status of coitarche), with cervical cytology testing exclusively until 30 years old.
- For woman 30 to 65 years of age, co-testing with HPV and cytology testing every five years is the preferred method of screening. Cytology screening every three years.
- Discontinue screening for women over the age of 65 without a history of cervical intraepithelial neoplasia (CIN) grade 2 or higher and for who have had adequate prior negative screening results.
- Woman with history of CIN2 or higher shouldn't be screened for 20 years following the initial post-treatment surveillance period, regardless of whether or not they have had a full hysterectomy.

The Bethesda System was developed to standardize the cytological findings on Pap smears. In 2001 there was a revision, with a few changes. Below, it is the classification of abnormalities in squamous and glandular epithelium.

According to the Bethesda System (TBS) 2001 [13]:
Squamous epithelium:

- Atypical squamous cells
  - Atypical squamous cells of the undertermined significance (ASC-US)
  - Atypical squamous cells the - cannot exclude HSIL (ASC-H)

- Low-grade squamous intraepithelial lesion (LSIL or LGSIL)
- High-grade squamous intraepithelial lesion (HSIL or HGSIL)
- Squamous cell carcinoma

Glandular epithelium:

- Atypical Glandular Cells not otherwise specified (AGC-NOS)
- Atypical Glandular Cells, suspicious for AIS or cancer (AGC-neoplastic)
- Adenocarcinoma in situ (AIS).

Cytological Abnormalities in Squamous Cell

The milder abnormalities in squamous cell are represented by the ASC-US and LSIL classification. They may be from transient lesions to low grade squamous intraepithelial lesions (CIN1/HPV). These injuries are mostly caused by HPV, but one should always discard local infections by other agents and inflammatory changes. There is a small chance of progression to more severe dysplasia (12-16%), bearing is indicated colposcopy with directed biopsies for anatomopathological study [14].

Cytological lesions classified as ASC-H and HSIL are more severe dysplasias suggesting moderate to severe intraepithelial neoplasia or carcinoma in situ. It may progress to invasive cancer if not treated properly.

These cytological abnormalities present are indicative of colposcopy to perform targeted biopsies, material is sent to pathology for diagnostic confirmation by histology [14].

Repeat cytology is an option for women with abnormal cervical citology. Reflex HPV testing (HPV test used after an inconclusive Pap test) is another acceptable conduct in ASC-US management [15]. The referral to colposcopy only of patients with high-risk HPV positive is a possible option.

Colposcopic Findings in Squamous Lesions

The classification of colposcopic findings was organized in a consensus in 2011, by the *International Federation of Cervical Pathology and Colposcopy Colposcopic*, as shown below [16]:

TERMINOLOGY OF THE CERVIX

- General Assessment
  - Adequate or inadequate for the reason (eg. cervix obscured by inflammation, bleeding, scar)
  - Squamocolumnar junction visibility: completely visible, partially visible, not visible
  - Transformation zone types 1, 2, 3
- Normal Colposcopic Findings
  - Original squamous epithelium: mature, atrophic
  - Columnar epithelium; ectopy/ectropion
  - Metaplastic squamous epithelium; Nabothian cysts; crypt (gland) opening
  - Deciduosis in pregnancy
- Abnormal Findings Colposcopic
  - Location of the lesion: inside or outside the transformation zone; location of the lesion by clock position
  - Size of the lesion: number of cervical quadrants the lesion covers
  - Size of the lesion percentage of the cervix
  - Grade 1 (minor)
    o Fine mosaic; fine punctation, thin acetowhite epithelium; irregular, geographic border
  - Grade 2 (major)
    o Sharp border; inner border sign; dense acetowhite epithelium; coarse mosaic; coarse punctation; rapid appearance of acetowhitening, cuffed crypt (gland) openings
- Nonspecific

- Leukoplakia (keratosis, hyperkeratosis), erosion
- Lugol's staining (Schiller's test): stained or nonstained
- Suspicious for invasion
  - Atypical vessels
  - Additional signs: fragile vessels, irregular surface, exophytic lesion, necrosis, ulceration, tumor or neoplasm gross
- Miscellaneous findings
  - Congenital transformation zone, condyloma, polyp, inflammation, stenosis, congenital anormaly, posttreatment consequence, endometriosis

Colposcopy with directed biopsies is described as gold standard for the diagnosis of cervical precancerous lesions. Colposcopy has a sensitivity ranging from 87% to 99% to diagnose cervical neoplasia, but its specificity is lower, between 23% and 87% [17, 18].

Protocols for embodiments of colposcopy are still somewhat controversial. However, it can be said that there are three main directions: biopsy of the worst-appearing lesion if the lesion is observed, biopsy several of acetowhite lesions, and strategies involving random biopsies of the normal-appearing epithelium in four quadrants [19].

The colposcopic findings suggest that tissue changes include: color tone of acetowhite areas, borderline between acetowhite areas and the rest of the epithelium; vascular features and color changes after application of iodine [20].

VASCULAR CHANGES

The local vascular distribution should be assessed before the application of acetic acid to the search punctation, mosaics and atypical vessels. These abnormalities are suggestive of local injury.

The capillaries usually are restricted to vessels in immature metaplasia region and form a fine network below the basement membrane. When there is formation of CIN, this network is incorporated into the dysplastic epithelium, and finely covered with a thin tissue layer. Venous endings displaying shaped punctations and the vessels running parallel to the surface are displayed as mosaics. Punctations and mosaics can be classified as fine or course. Punctations are fine capillary endings of small diameter, grouped. Fine mosaics are networks with small diameter capillaries, grouped, arranged parallel to the surface. These changes are commonly viewed in low-grade lesions. Coarse punctation and coarse mosaics are capillary formations of higher caliber and more remote. They are more common in severe dysplasia [20].

LEUKOPLAKIA

The leukoplakia is a lesion formed by keratin. It can be idiopathic, caused by chronic infection and even HPV. It is a white, well-defined area in the cervix that can be viewed with the naked eye, prior to application of acetic acid. Wherever displayed, should be biopsied for correct diagnosis [20].

CONDYLOMATA

It is an exophytic lesion, sometimes found in the transformation zone. They can be multiple and of varying sizes and can also be seen with the naked eye. In colposcopy, has a central capillary and irregular appearance (brainlike texture). Usually it does not stain with the application of iodine and should always be biopsied when viewed [20].

APPLICATION OF ACETIC ACID

Acetic acid acts by reversibly coagulates nuclear proteins. Areas where there is a greater number of mitosis/cell division have stronger reaction during application of this reagent. Therefore, the acetic acid leads to highlight the areas where there is likely to neoplastic lesion. There is a direct correlation in the intensity of the dull, white color, effect duration, and severity of the injury. The higher the degree of dysplasia, the more pronounced is the effect.

Low-grade CIN lesions are less dense, less extensive and less complex acetowhite areas, compared with high-grade CIN lesions. They tend to be thin, may have fine punctations and fine mosaics. They are farther away from the squamocolumnar junction when compared to high-grade lesions [21, 22].

High-grade lesions, in contrast, have dense acetowhite areas, well-defined, with lasting reaction on the application of acetic acid. Are more complex and extensive lesions, can enter the endocervical canal. These findings have less glare, usually occupy the two lips of the cervix and can lead to cervical obliteration.

The surface of high-grade lesions may become irregular, nodular compared to the surrounding epithelium. Glandular crypts, common in Transformation zone may show thickening and halo, called cuffed crypt openings.

The main differences between low and high grade squamous intraepithelial lesions include the density and definition colposcopic images, being more intense in the last.

Acetowhite staining is not pathognomonic of intraepithelial lesion. It can be physiological in areas of cell metaplasia, and can also be present in inflammations. Acetowhite epithelium is suggestive of cancer when found in the transformation zone, the squamocolumnar junction, well defined compared to normal epithelium around them [20].

APPLICATION OF LUGOL'S IODINE SOLUTION (SCHILLER'S TEST)

The existing squamous epithelium in the cervix and vaginal walls, and also in areas of metaplasia show glycogen-rich cells. Glycogen is stained brown or black by lugol's iodine solution. In dysplasic/neoplastic tissues, glycogen is at a low level due to heavy consumption during mitosis. During the application of the reagent, these areas do not stain or partially stain (mustard or saffron yellow colors). Atrophic epithelia (postmenopausal women) and condyloma lesions do not stain (or stain partially) after administration of the reagent.

According to these findings, the colposcopist can suggest the diagnosis by the intensity of colposcopic findings, but the definitive diagnosis will be made after biopsy:

- Normal (Negative)
- Low-grade CIN
- High-grade CIN
- Invasive Cancer
- Other (eg inflammation)

- Unsatisfactory colposcopy (eg squamocolumnar junction not displayed)

ADENOCARCINOMA

Endocervical adenocarcinoma is the second most common type of cervical malignancy [21], corresponding to approximately 20% of cervical cancers [21, 22].The natural history of adenocarcinoma is similar to squamous cell carcinoma, particularly in relation to the existence of precursor lesions and association with HPV infection of high oncogenic risk [21].

Less than 1% of Pap smears results are diagnosed as atypical glandular cells [23, 24]. The atypical glandular cells findings are divided by the final qualifying Bethesda (2001) in atypical glandular cells of undetermined significance (AGC), adenocarcinoma in situ and invasive adenocarcinoma of the cervix [21]. The interpretation of AGC must be qualified if possible to indicate whether the cells would be of endocervical or endometrial origin;if the source of the cells can not be determined, we use the generic term "glandular" [13]. The AGC category was further divided into unspecified atypical glandular cells (NOS) and AGC possibly neoplastic [21].

The cervical cytology is primarily a screening test for squamous intraepithelial lesions and squamous cell carcinoma.Sensitivity to the glandular lesions is limited by problems with the sample and its interpretation [25, 26] and compared with squamous cell cancer, cytology has been relatively ineffective in decreasing incidence of invasive adenocarcinoma of the cervix [27]. The glandular smear tends to be problematic because the glandular lesions usually occur deep inside neck of the glands of the uterus or the endocervical canal [24, 26]. The low prevalence of AGC in cervical cytology, the relative absence of findings on colposcopy and a wide range of differential diagnosis are factors that represent a significant diagnostic challenge for cytopathologists and clinical trials [21]. Some studies have suggested an increased incidence of cervical adenocarcinoma, which may be a consequence of the relatively low ability to detect glandular lesions screening techniques of the cervical cancers [26].

Women with atypical glandular cells on Pap smears were correlated with a high risk of clinically significant injuries, including invasive cancer [26]. There is consensus in the literature and in medical practice indicating the colposcopy with biopsy guided as first choice in patients with alterations in Pap smear, even in smears with atypical glandular cells [7, 22, 23, 24, 28].

However other options are also described, such as endocervical curettage [29] or endometrial [24] and currently the HPV DNA research [21, 26, 27, 30].

The colposcopy is a subjective test and its diagnostic accuracy has been questioned for decades [28]. In cases of endocervical glandular lesions and premalignant lesions, the benefit of colposcopy is very challenged by the difficulty in visualization of the lesion and identifying areas for performing biopsy.Few studies correlate the AGC cytology with abnormal colposcopic findings. Some studies suggest the performance of endocervical curettage in the initial evaluation of smears with atypical glandular [29], especially in women with colposcopy unsatisfactory for not viewing the squamou-colunnar junction over 40 years [28, 29], however this procedure remains controversial [29].

We know the technical difficulty of colposcopy examination to identify endocervical lesions that are usually hidden inside the endocervical canal and therefore the value of HPV testing in the clinical management of women with this cytological diagnosis has received attention in recent years [21]. HPV DNA research has very important role in cases of AGC [21] as often exhibit significant correlation with clinically significant injuries, including invasive adenocarcinoma by identifying those most at risk of occult lesions.

Whereas the high-risk HPV testing is widely accepted in screening of women with atypical squamous lesions [31, 32] its role in patients with AGC is not fully elucidated [33].

In the United States and most of Europe, the recommendation to increase the HPV test use in screening, post colposcopy and after treatment seems to help enhance early diagnosis of pre cancerous lesions and adenocarcinoma in situ compared with isolated cytology [30]. Several ways are described for the introduction of HPV testing in treating patients with AGC.The 2012 consensus guidelines of the American Society for Colposcopy and Cervical Pathology established that the addition of HPV testing to cytology improved the identification of women with cervical adenocarcinoma and its precursor lesions [27]. Thus, the increase in the combined use of cytology and HPV (cotesting) may lower failure rates with respect to glandular lesions [26].

The HPV testing can also be performed at the time of colposcopy examination and some studies show that this can be a powerful auxiliary tool for identifying women at high risk of significant cervical lesions underlying, especially where not found any colposcopy abnormality [21].

POST-TREATMENT

Current clinical guidelines recommend Pap smear in the first 5 years after surgical treatment of CIN (conization, loop electrosurgical excision or large loop excision of the transformation zone), which can be accompanied by colposcopy [34]. This follow-up can vary from quarterly to semi-annual, depending on the guideline used. The recurrence rates after treatment of CIN range from 5 to 10% [35, 36, 37, 38]. Therefore, there is the concern to hold a closed follow-up.

There are some predictor factors that are associated with increased risk of recurrence, such as the presence of positive margins [39], age greater than 50 years to treatment [40], pretreatment viral load [41] and multiparity [42]. An important cause of residual or recurrent disease is HPV persistence [41, 43].

The association of Pap smear with HPV testing (cotesting) would be a good option in the follow-up post-treatment of CIN 2 and CIN 3 [44, 45]. If the surgical margins of the surgical procedure were negative and the patient has negative cotesting at 6 and 12 month follow-up, 18 months visit could be avoided, and new test could be accomplished in five years [46]. Another option is to perform cotesting at 6 and 24 months post-treatment, and if negative, the patient would be retested only 5 years later [41, 47].

In countries where the public health system has no available HPV testing, and when the HPV testing is positive, the colposcopy is an important test for viewing changes and perform directed cervical biopsy, setting the correct diagnosis of recurrence and treatment.

CONCLUSION

The colposcopy has great value in detecting cervical mucosa abnormalities and it is an essential test for biopsy, which is the gold standard for detection of premalignant and malignant cervical lesions. Diagnostic accuracy depends largely on clinical experience. The advent of molecular testing for HPV led to changes in the conduct of referrals to colposcopy, which does not diminish the importance of the colposcopy. Thus, the combination of colposcopy and HPV testing is a potential alternative for improved diagnosis of cervical lesions.

REFERENCES

[1]   Benedet, J.L.; Anderson, G.H.; Boyes, D.A. 1985. "Colposcopic accuracy in the diagnosis of microinvasive and occult invasive carcinoma of the cervix." *Obstet. Gynecol.* 65(4):557–62.

[2]   Sideri, M.; Garutti, P.; Costa, S.; Cristiani, P.; Schincaglia, P.; Sassoli de Bianchi, P.; Naldoni, C.; Bucchi, L. 2015. "Accuracy of Colposcopically Directed Biopsy: Results from an Online Quality Assurance Programme for Colposcopy in a Population-Based Cervical Screening Setting in Italy." *Biomed. Res. Int.* 2015:614035.

[3]   Kierkegaard, O.; Byrjalsen, C.; Frandsen, K.H.; Hansen, KC; Frydenberg, M. 1994. "Diagnostic accuracy of cytology and colposcopy in cervical squamous intraepithelial lesions." *Acta Obstet. Gynecol Scand.* 73 (8):648–51.

[4]   Torre, L.A.; Bray, F.; Siegel, R.L.; Ferlay, J.; Lortet-Tieulent, J.; Jemal, A. 2015. "Global cancer statistics, 2012." *CA Cancer J. Clin.* 65(2):87-108.

[5]   U.S. Cancer Statistics Working Group. 2015. United States Cancer Statistics: 1999–2012 Incidence and Mortality Web-based Report. Atlanta (GA): Department of Health and Human Services, Centers for Disease Control and Prevention, and National Cancer Institute.

[6]   Wu, T.; Cheung, T.H.; Yim, S.F.; Qu, J.Y. 2010. "Clinical study of quantitative diagnosis of early cervical cancer based on the classification of acetowhitening kinetics." *J. Biomed. Opt.* 15(2):026001.

[7]   Davies, K.R.; Cantor, S.B.; Cox, D.D.; Follen, M. 2015. "An Alternative Approach for Estimating the Accuracy of Colposcopy in Detecting Cervical Precancer." *PLoS One.* 10(5):e0126573.

[8]   Karjane, N. & Chelmow, D. 2013. "New Cervical Cancer Screening Guidelines, Again." *Obstet. Gynecol. Clin. North Am.* 40(2):211-23.

[9]   Franco, E.L. 2003. "Chapter 13: Primary screening of cervical cancer with human papillomavirus tests." *J. Natl. Cancer Inst. Monogr.*; (31):89-96.

[10] Nomelini, R.S.; Barcelos, A.C.; Michelin, M.A.; Adad, S.J.; Murta, E.F. 2007. "Utilization of human papillomavirus testing for cervical cancer prevention in a university hospital." *Cad. Saude Publica.* 23(6):1309-18.

[11] Nomelini, R.S.; Guimarães, P.D.; Candido, P.A.; Campos, A.C.; Michelin, M.A.; Murta, E.F. 2012. "Prevention of cervical cancer in women with ASCUS in the Brazilian Unified National Health System:

cost-effectiveness of the molecular biology method for HPV detection." *Cad Saude Publica*. 28(11):2043-52.

[12] Schiffman, M. & Solomon, D. 2013. "Cervical-cancer screening with human papillomavirus and cytologic cotesting." *N. Engl. J. Med.* 369:2324–2331.

[13] Solomon, D. & Nayar, R. 2004. *The Bethesda System for Roporten Cervical Citology – Definitions, Criteria, and Explanatory Nots*. New York: Springer-Verlag.

[14] Schlichte, M.J. & Guidry, J. 2015. "Current Cervical Carcinoma Screening Guidelines." *J. Clin. Med.* 7;4(5):918-32.

[15] Massad, L.S.; Einstein, M.H.; Huh, W.K.; Katki, H.A.; Kinney, W.K.; Schiffman, M.; Solomon, D.; Wentzensen, N.; Lawson, H.W.; 2012 ASCCP Consensus Guidelines Conference. "2012 updated consensus guidelines for the management of abnormal cervical cancer screening tests and cancer precursors." *J. Low Genit Tract. Dis.* 2013; 17:S1–27.

[16] Bornstein, J.; Bentley, J.; Bösze, P.; Girardi, F.; Haefner, H.; Menton, M.; Perrotta, M.; Prendiville, W.; Russell, P.; Sideri, M.; Strander, B.; Tatti, S.; Torne, A.; Walker, P. 2012. "2011 colposcopic terminology of the International Federation for Cervical Pathology and Colposcopy." *Obstet. Gynecol.* 120(1):166-72.

[17] Mitchell, M.F.; Cantor, S.B.; Ramanujam, N.; Tortolero-Luna, G.; Richards-Kortum, R. 1999. "Fluorescence spectroscopy for diagnosis of squamous intraepithelial lesions of the cervix." *Obstet. Gynecol.* 93:462-70.

[18] Belinson, J.L.; Pretorius, R.G.; Zhang, W.H.; Wu, L.Y.; Qiao, Y.L.; Elson, P. 2001."Cervical cancer screening by simple visual inspection after acetic acid." *Obstet. Gynecol.* 98(3):441-4.

[19] Schiffman, M. & Wentzensen, N. 2015. "Issues in optimising and standardising the accuracy and utility of the colposcopic examination in the HPV era." *Ecancermedicalscience*. 29; 9:530.

[20] Sellors, J.W. & Sankaranarayanan, R.. International Agency for Research on Cancer. Colposcopy and treatment of cervical intraepithelial neoplasia: a beginner's manual. England: M J Webb Associates, Newmarket, printed in France.

[21] Zeferino, L.C.; Rabelo-Santos, S. H.; Villa, L. L.; Sarian, L. O.; Costa, M. C.; Westin, M.C.A.; Ângelo-Andrade, A.L.; Derchain, S. 2011. "Value of HPV-DNA test in women with cytological diagnosis of atypical glandular cells (AGC)." *European Journal of Obstetrics & Gynecology and Reproductive Biology 159:* 160-164.

[22] Partridge, E. E.; Abu-Rustum, N.; Giuliano, A.; Massad, S.; McClure, J.; Dwyer, M.; Hughes, M. 2014. "Cervical Cancer Screening – Featured Updates." *Journal of the National Comprehensive Cancer Network* 12(3):333-341.

[23] Schorge, J. O. & Rauh-Hain, J. A. 2013. "Atypical Glandular cells." *Clinical Obstetrics and Gynecology* 56(1)35-43.

[24] Munro, A.; Williams, V.; Semmens, J.; Leung, Y.; Stewart, C. J.; Codde, J.; Spilsbury, K.; Steel, N.; Cohen, P.; O'Leary, P. 2015. "Risk of high grade Cervical dysplasia and gynaecological malignancies following the cytologic diagnosis of atypical endocervical cells of undeterminade significance: A Retrospective study of a state-wide screening population in Western Australia." *Australian and New Zealand Journal of Obstetrics and Gynaecology* 55:268-273.

[25] Moriarty, A. T. & Wilbur, D. 2003. "Those gland problems in cervical cytology: faith ou fact? Observations from the Bethesda 2001 terminology conference" *Diagnostic Cytopathology 8(4):*171-174.

[26] Miller, R. A.; Mody, D. R.; Tams, K. C.; Thrall, M. J. 2015. "Glandular lesions of the cervix in Clinical Practice – A Citology, histology and human papillomavirus correlation study from 2 institutions." *Archives of Pathology & Laboratory Medicine* 139(11):1431-1436.

[27] Saslow, D.; Solomon, D.; Lawson, H. W.; Killackey, M.; Kulasingem, S. L.; Cain, J.; Garcia, F.A.R., Moriarty, A.T.; Waxman, A.G.; Wilbur, D.C.; Wentzensen, N.; Downs, L.S. J.; Spitzer, M.; Moscicki, A.; Franco, E. L.; Stoler, M. H.; Schiffman, M.; Castle, P. E.; Myers, E. R. 2012. "American Cancer Society, American Society for Colposcopy and Cervical Pathology, and American Society for Clinical Pathology Screening Guidelines for the Prevention and Early Detection of Cervical Cancer." *A Cancer Journal for Clinicians* 62:147-172.

[28] Nakamura, Y.; Matsumoto, K.; Satoh, T.; Nishide, K.; Nozue, A.; Shimabukuro, K.; Endo, S.; Nagai, K.; Oki, A.; Minaguchi, T.; Morishita, Y.; Noguchi, M.; Yoshikawa, H. 2015. "Optimising biopsy procedures during colposcopy for women with abnormal cervical cancer screening results: a multicenter prospective study." Internacional Journal of Clinical Oncology 20:579-585.

[29] Apgar, B. S.; Kaufman, A. J.; Bettcher, C.; Parker-Featherstone, E. 2013. "Gynecologic Procedures: Colposcopy treatment of cervical Intraepithelialneoplasia, and Endometrial Assessment." *American Family Physician* 80(12):836-843.

[30] Waxman, A. G. 2013. "Cervical Cancer Prevention. New Guidelines in the United States and New opportunities for Low and Middle-Income Countries." *Obstetrics & Gynecology Clinics of North America* 251-255.

[31] Prendiville, W. 2005. "Recent innovations in colposcopy practice." *Best Practice & Research Clinical Obstetrics and Gynaecoogy* 5:779-792.

[32] Castle, P. E.; Eaton, B.; Reid, J.; Getman, D.; Dockter, J. 2015. "Comparison of Human Papillomavirus Detection by Aptima HPV and cobas HPV Tests in a Population of Women referred for Colposcopy following Detection of Atypical Squamous Cells of Undetermined Significance by Pap Cytology." *Journal of Clinical Microbiology* 53:1277-1281.

[33] Verdoodt, F.; Jiang, X.; Williams, M.; Schnatz, P. F.; Arbyn, M. 2015. Hight-risk HPV testing in the management of atypical glandular cells: A Systematic review and meta-analysis. *International Journal of cancer*. In Press.

[34] Colposcopy and programme management: guidelines for the NHS cervical screening programme. NHSCSP publication no. 20; 2004.

[35] Dobbs, S.P.; Asmussen, T.; Nunns, D.; Hollingworth, J.; Brown, L.J.; Ireland, D. 2000. "Does histological incomplete excision of cervical intraepithelial neoplasia following large loop excision of transformation zone increase recurrence rates? A six year cytological follow up." *Br. J. ObstetGynaecol.* 107: 1298–1301.

[36] Bigrigg, M.A.; Codling, B.W.; Pearson, P.; Read, M.D.; Swingler GR. 1990. "Colposcopic diagnosis and treatment of cervical dysplasia at a single clinic visit." *Lancet* 306: 229–231.

[37] Chew, G.K.; Jandial, L.; Paraskevaidis, E.; Kitchener, H.C. 1999. "Pattern of CIN recurrence following laser ablation treatment on long term follow up." *Int. J. Gynecol. Cancer* 9: 487–490.

[38] Flannelly, G.; Langhan, H.; Jandial, L.; Mana, E.; Campbell., M; Kitchener, H. 1997. "A study of treatment failures following large loop excision of the transformation zone for the treatment of cervical intraepithelial neoplasia." *Br. J. Obstet. Gynaecol.* 104:718–722.

[39] Gardeil, F.; Barry Walsh, C.; Prendiville, W.; Clinch, J.; Turner, M.J. 1997. "Persistent intraepithelial neoplasia after excision for cervical intraepithelial neoplasia grade III." *Obstet. Gynaecol.* 89: 419–422.

[40] Fogle, R.H.; Spann, CO; Easley, K.A.; Basil, J.B. 2004. "Predictors of cervical dysplasia after the loop electrosurgical excision procedure in an inner-city population." *J. Reprod. Med.* 49(6):481-6.49.

[41] Mo, L.Z.; Song, H.L.; Wang, J.L.; He, Q.; Qiu, Z.C.; Li, F. 2015. "Pap Smear Combined with HPV Testing: A Reasonable Tool for Women with High-grade Cervical Intraepithelial Neoplasia Treated by LEEP." *Asian Pac. J. Cancer Prev.* 16(10):4297-302.

[42] Liu, W.J.; Liu, X.S.; Zhao, K.N.; Leggatt, G.R.; Frazer, I.H. 2000. "Papillomavirus virus-like particles for the delivery of multiple cytotoxic t-cell epitopes." *Virology* 273: 374–382.

[43] Du, R.; Meng, W.; Chen, Z.F.; Zhang, Y.; Chen, S.Y.; Ding, Y. 2013. "Post-treatment human papillomavirus status and recurrence rates in patients treated with loop electrosurgical excision procedure conization for cervical intraepithelial neoplasia." *Eur. J. GynaecolOncol.* 34(6):548-51.

[44] Agapova, M.; Duignan, A.; Smith, A.; O'Neill, C.; Basu A. 2015. "Long-term costs of introducing HPV-DNA post-treatment surveillance to national cervical cancer screening in Ireland." *Expert Rev. Pharmacoecon Outcomes Res.* 17:1-7.

[45] Costa, S.; Venturoli, S.; Origoni, M.; Preti, M.; Mariani, L.; Cristoforoni, P.; Sandri, M.T. 2015. "Performance of HPV DNA testing in the follow-up after treatment of high-grade cervical lesions, adenocarcinoma in situ (AIS) and microinvasive carcinoma." *Ecancermedicalscience* 29; 9:528.

[46] Ruano, Y.; Torrents, M.; Ferrer, F.J. 2015. "Human papillomavirus combined with cytology and margin status identifies patients at risk for recurrence after conization for high-grade cervical intraepithelial neoplasia." *Eur. J. Gynaecol. Oncol.* 36(3):245-51.

[47] Uijterwaal, M.H.; Kocken, M.; Berkhof, J.; Bekkers, R.L.; Verheijen, R.H.; Helmerhorst, T.J.; Meijer C.J. 2014. "Posttreatment assessment of women at risk of developing high-grade cervical disease: proposal for new guidelines based on data from the Netherlands." *J. Low Genit Tract. Dis.* 18(4):338-43.

In: Cryosurgery and Colposcopy
Editor: Lillian Watson

ISBN: 978-1-63484-507-6
© 2016 Nova Science Publishers, Inc.

Chapter 4

DIAGNOSIS AND MANAGEMENT OF VAGINAL INTRAEPITHELIAL NEOPLASIA

Laurie Elit*, MD, MSc, FRCS(C)
Division of Gynecologic Oncology,
Department of Obstetrics and Gynecology, McMaster University,
Hamilton, Canada

ABSTRACT

Vaginal Intraepithelial Neoplasia (VaIN) is a rare preinvasive disease that accounts for up to 1% of women who attend the colposcopy clinic. In this chapter we will review the characteristics of the disease (i.e., location in the vagina, single versus multifocal presentation), the risk factors for VaIN (i.e., other invasive or pre-invasive disease of the low genital tract, smoking), methods of screening for the diagnosis (including vaginal cytology, oncHPV testing), and role of colposcopy in making the diagnosis. Strategies for enhancing the colposcopic identification of VaIN will be discussed such as the use of vaginal estrogen, use of 3-5% acetic acid and Lugol's solution.

Treatment strategies, indications for specific maneuvers and the likelihood of success and complications will be presented for 5FU (Effudex®), CO_2 laser ablation/excision, upper vaginectomy, colpectomy, vaginal brachytherapy, and Aldara®. Recommendations for follow-up will be provided.

---

* elitlor@hhsc.ca.

ABBREVIATIONS

CIN	Cervical Intraepithelial neoplasia
CUSA	Cavitational Ultrasonic surgical aspiration
DES	Diethylstilbesterol
HG VaIN	High Grade Vaginal Intraepithelial Neoplasia (Grades 2-3)
HPV	Human Papilloma Virus
HR HPV	High Risk Human Papilloma Virus (oncogenic HPV)
HIV	Human Immunodeficiency virus
LAST	lower anogenital squamous terminology
LEEP	Loop electrosurgical Procedure
LGT	Lower Genital Tract
LGT IN	Lower Genital Tract intraepithelial neoplasia
LG VaIN	Low Grade Vaginal Intraepithelial Neoplasia (Grade 1)
Y-PGA	Poly-Y-glutamic acid
VaIN 1	Vaginal Intraepithelial Neoplasia grade 1
VaIN 2	Vaginal Intraepithelial Neoplasia grade 2
VaIN 3	Vaginal Intraepithelial Neoplasia grade 3
5FU	5 Flurouracil

INTRODUCTION

In 2008, there were 13,000 new vaginal cancers globally. Thus 2% of gynecologic cancers are vaginal cancer making vaginal cancer quite rare [1]. To put this in context for the United States in 2014, 4,700 women were affected with vaginal cancer and 910 died of this disease [2]. Similar to cervical cancer, vaginal cancer is preceded by a preinvasive form of disease known as vaginal intra-epithelial neoplasia (VaIN). VaIN was first described by Hummer in 1933 [3].

Graham and Meigs first described VaIN in the American literature in 1952 [4]. Prevention of vaginal cancer is by vaccination prior to coital exposure of oncogenic HPV or through identification and treatment of VaIN usually through a cervical cancer prevention program. In this chapter, we will discuss the nomenclature, epidemiology, risk factors, strategies to identify, treatment options and follow-up strategies for VaIN.

METHODS

A literature search was conducted from 2000-Jun 2015 using PubMed and Google. Search terms included: vaginal intra-epithelial neoplasia, vaginal dysplasia. All articles including case reports, case series, cohort studies, randomized trials and meta-analyses were reviewed.

Nomenclature

As with terminology for cervical intraepithelial neoplasia (CIN), there is VaIN grades 1, 2 and 3. VaIN is defined as the presence of squamous cell atypia without stromal invasion. In VaIN 1, the lower one-third of vaginal epithelial is involved (See Figure 1 and 2). In VaIN 2, the lower two-third of vaginal epithelial is involved. In VaIN 3, more than two thirds of vaginal epithelial is involved (See Figure 3 and 4). One of the problems encountered with this classification system is the lack of intra and inter pathologists reproducibility of the histologic diagnosis.

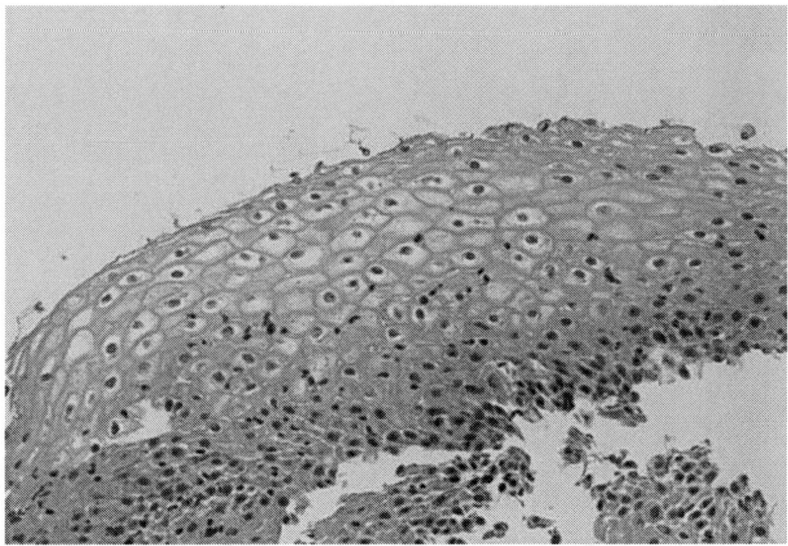

Figure 1. VaIN 1 Normal vaginal epithelium. Photograph by Jennifer Michelle Dmetrichuk.

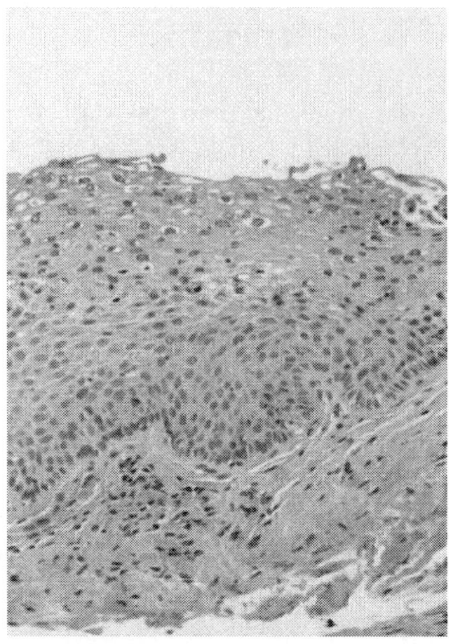

Figure 2. VaIN 1. Dysplastic cells make up the lower one third of the epithelium. Photograph by Jennifer Michelle Dmetrichuk.

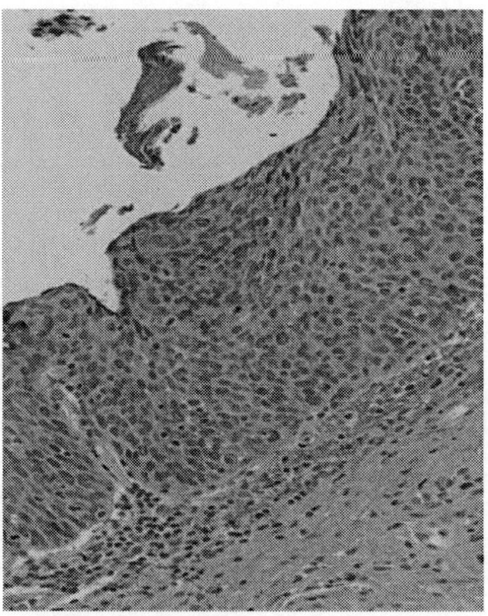

Figure 3. VaIN 3. Dysplastic cells replace the whole epithelium. Photograph by Jennifer Michelle Dmetrichuk.

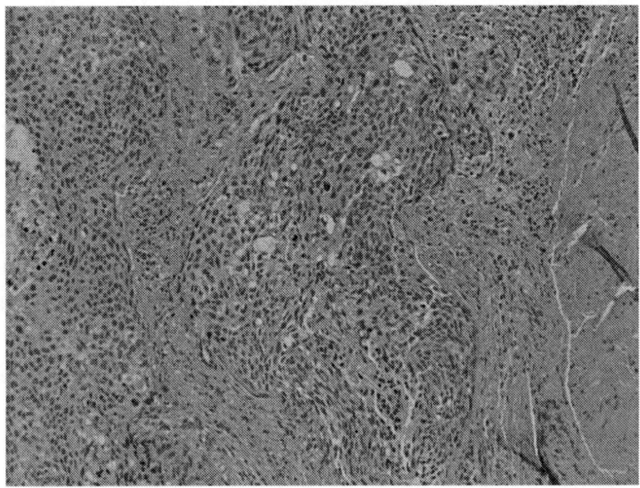

Figure 4. Squamous cell carcinoma. Photograph by Jennifer Michelle Dmetrichuk.

The lower anogenital squamous terminology (LAST) standardization project for human papilloma virus (HPV) associated lesions categories as put forward by the College of American Pathologists and American Society of Colposcopy and Cervical Pathology have proposed revised terminology. They have recommended to call VaIN 1-low grade and VaIN 2/3 -high grade squamous intraepithelial lesion (LSIL, HSIL) [5].

Intraepitheial vaginal dysplasia of glandular origin or atypical vaginal adenosis is a separate entity. Although usually associated with exposure to in utero diethylstilbestrol (DES) [5] there have been atypical adenosis cases associated with vaginal adenocarcinoma in non-DES exposed women [5].

INCIDENCE AND PREVALENCE

The incidence of VaIN is 0.2 per 100,000 women [6]. It accounts for 0.4% of intraepithelial disease in the lower genital tract [6, 7, 8] or in other words is 100-fold less common than CIN. Rates of VaIN appear to be increasing as a result of increased awareness, cytology screening and more widespread use of colposcopy [7]. One of the questions is why VaIN is so rare compared to the high prevalence of CIN? The mature stable squamous epithelium of the vagina is less vulnerable to the effects of HPV on epithelial such as the metaplastic transformation zone of the cervix [6].

Natural History

What happens to VaIN if it is not treated? Aho in 1991 [9] described 23 women with VaIN who were not treated but were followed for 3 years. Of these 23, two (9%) progressed to invasive cancer, 3 (13%) had persistent VaIN and 18 (78%) regressed. Regress was less likely if both the cervix and vagina were involved (67% versus 91%). These rates of progression are less than seen with CIN. It is hypothesized that the mature stable squamous epithelium of the vagina is less vulnerable to the effects of HPV compared to that of the metaplastic transformation zone of the cervix [6].

One of the complex issues with the diagnosis of VaIN 3 is that it may actually represent invasive cancer. Bornstein [10] described 32 women who had an upper vaginectomy for VaIN 3 and 9 (28%) already had an underlying invasive cancer.

Risk Factors

Risk factors for vaginal cancer and VaIN are similar to those of cervical cancer. These include: smoking [1, 4, 6, 11], genetic or acquired immunosuppression [1, 6, 8], and the high number of sexual partners [1]. Risk factors unique to vaginal cancer and VaIN include: history of cervical precancers and cancers [1, 8, 12] or neoplasia or cervix or vulva [6] or vulvar dysplasia [4], cervical dysplasia treated by hysterectomy [6, 8, 12], prior pelvic radiation [8, 12], and increasing age especially over 60 years [8]. Evidence for these risk factors is outlined below.

Age: The average age of women diagnosed with VaIN is 43-60 yo with a peak of 70-79 years.

Smoking: Sherman [13] showed in 111 women (71 with HG VaIN and 40 with LG VaIN) that 41% had a smoking history. Women who were smokers and had HR-HPV were at higher risk of HG VaIN compared to nonsmokers (83% vs 59%, p = 0.02)

Immunosuppression: Massad [14] showed in 335 seropositive HIV women and 75 seronegative women with prior hysterectomy that the risk of VaIN was 0.2 per 100 person years in those who were seropositive and 0.1 per 100 person years for those who were seronegative (p = 0.001).

Lower genital tract Neoplasia: About 50% of VaIN cases share the same HPV profile as the other LGT infections [6, 15], there were 49 cases of cervical cancer with synchronous CIN and VaIN. In 58.7% of these cases the HPV genotype was the same in all three locations.

Hysterectomy for CIN: VaIN occurs in 0.91% of women who had a hysterectomy for CIN 3 [6]. Schockaert [16] showed a rate of VaIN of 7.4% after hysterectomy for CIN. 7/94 women developed VaIN 2+ a median of 35 months (5-103 mos) after hysterectomy. In other words the risk of VaIN is 0.6/100,000 but can increase to 0.91% in women with a hysterectomy due to CIN gr 3 [17]. The reasons for VaIN after hysterectomy for CIN include: 1) unrecognized CIN extending to the vagina and not removed as part of the hysterectomy; and 2) if the VaIN occurs a long time after the hysterectomy, it could represent de nova VaIN.

Prior Radiation therapy: Li [18] looked at the impact of radiation on subsequent identification of VaIN and showed that compared 10 women who had had radiation compared to 23 women who had not had radiation, recurrence of VAIN 3 was higher in the radiated group (OR 3.625, 95% CI 1.454-9.0376). Time to recurrence was 12.3 months versus 15.3 months in controls. 3 and 1 women developed cancer respectively. VaIN in women who had had prior radiation was more refractory than in women how have VaIN without a history of radiation.

Evaluating the relative importance of various risk factors for VaIN, Li [19] conducted a case control study of 63 women with VaIN and 64 health controls. The risk factors for high grade VaIN by univariate analysis were pre or post-menopausal (2.09 95% CI 1.10-3.85, p = 0.024); prior hysterectomy (OR 4.69, p = 0.003); history of cervical cancer or CIN (OR 78.75, p < 0.0001), and HPV infection and high viral load (OR 125, p = 0.0001). In the multivariable analysis HPV infection and history of cervical cancer and CIN were important.

There is a unique form of vaginal cancer known as clear cell carcinoma that is related to in utero exposure to diethylstilbestrol (DES) that was used until 1970 as an abortive agent [1]. VaIN is not related to this form of vaginal cancer and so this clear cell cancer will not longer be discussed.

HPV

Oncologenic HPV is associated with vaginal cancer and VaIN. Alemany [1] conducted the largest and highest quality study in this regard.He used a highly sensitive SPG-10 polymerase chain reaction (PCR), DNA enzyme immunoassay (DEIA), HPV detection combined with LiPA 25 genotyping technique to assess 189 case of VaIN 2-3 and 408 cases of invasive vaginal cancers from 31 countries. The HPV DNA prevalence was 96% (95% CI 92-98%) in VaIN 2/3 and 74% (95%CI 70-78%) in vaginal cancers. High HPV prevalence was noted in younger women and those with squamous cell carcinomas with wary basaloid features. HPV 16 was found in 59% of VaIN 2-3, 6% HPV 18, 6% HPV 52, 5% HPV 73, 4% HPV 33, 4% HPV 59. Multiple HPV infections were seen in 11% of VaIN 2-3 cases. So showed in a different study that HPV load was higher in women with higher grades of VaIN [19] and persistent VaIN [20].

Diagnosis

Most women who present with VaIN are asymptomatic. The usual presentation is a woman who has had a hysterectomy for cervical dysplasia and has an abnormal post-hysterectomy follow-up Pap smear. Cheung [21] reported that 35.7% of cytology tests after hysterectomy for CIN are abnormal and in 19.6% VaIN is confirmed. This speaks to the importance of clearly documenting the extent of CIN prior to the hysterectomy so if an upper vaginectomy is required at the time of hysterectomy it is completed as one procedure. Some other presentations of VaIN include a woman who has symptoms like postcoital spotting or vaginal discharge.

Steps in the workup include a speculum examination of the vagina, vaginal cytology, digital palpation and colposcopy with biopsies. The colposcopic examination is conducted with 3-5% acetic acid with or without Lugol's solution. The most common finding is a raised or flat white lesion, but it could be granular in appearance with sharply demarcated borders (Figure 5) and rarely contact areas of vascular punctuation. The most common site for VaIN is the upper one-third of the vagina [12, 22]. This is a difficult area to visualize as the vaginal apices have redundancy and tunneling. A skin hook can be used to expose difficult to see areas. In those who have had a hysterectomy, the disease is often seen in the apices of the vault suture line [8, 11] report that 61% of women 121 with VaIN had multifocal disease. It is recommended to biopsy any acetowhite lesion, or a lesion that is Lugol's hypostaining (Figure 6, 7), or lesion with irregular surface. Excisional biopsy should be performed for an area of coarse vascular abnormality with unusual branching as this suggested invasive disease. The physical exam including vaginal palpation is usually conducted after the colposcopic exam. It may show areas of thickening or irregularity of the vaginal wall. The vaginal cuff should also be palpated.

If nothing is seen then the use of topical estrogen may accentuate subsequent visualization and improve detection of VaIN.

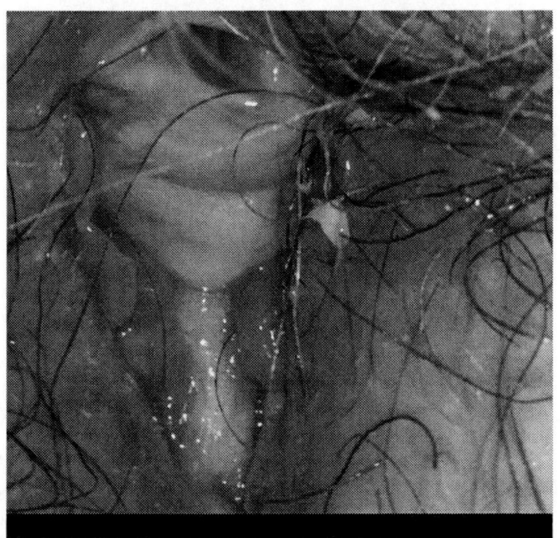

Figure 5. Aceto-white area in posterior vagina lower one third after application of 3% acetic acid. Photograph by Marrett Lee.

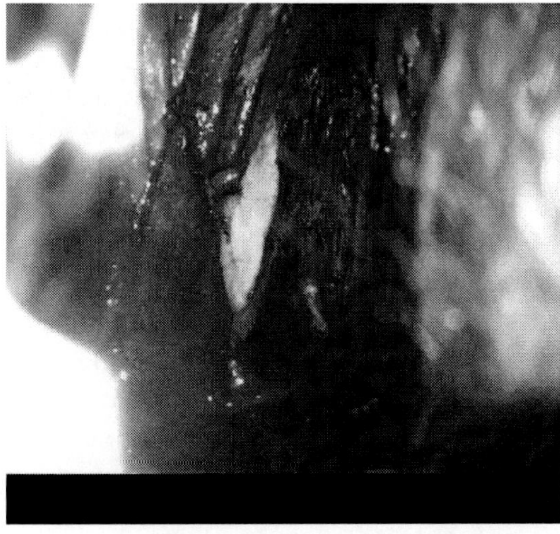

Figure 6. Lugol's absent area on the left lateral vagina. Photograph by Marrett Lee.

Laurie Elit

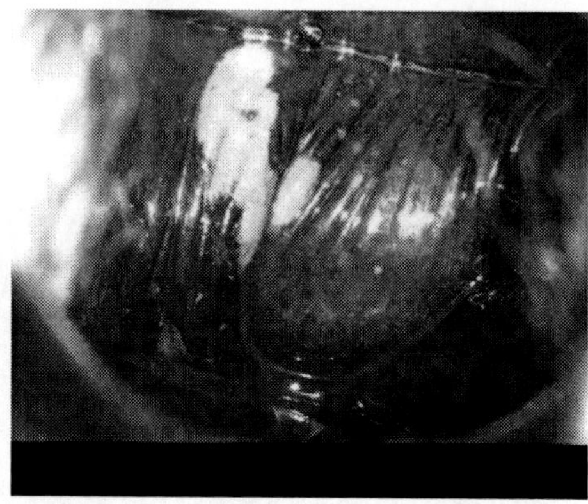

Figure 7. Lugol's absent area in the anterior vagina. Photograph by Marrett Lee.

Management

The treatment for VaIN should be individualized balancing the risk of disease persistence or recurrence with the need to minimize morbidity and preserve vaginal function [6]. Making this decision involves consideration of prior hysterectomy, prior radiation therapy, age, interest in preserving sexual activity, comorbidities and vaginal anatomy [7].

1. Observation

VaIN has been observed without medical or surgical treatment and it has been seen to regress. Aho 1991 followed 23 women with all grades of VaIN and showed a 78% regression rate, 13% persistence and 9% preogression to cancer. Situations where the disease is less likely to regress include association with cervical CIN (67% regression compared to 91% when no association with CIN) [6].

2. Treatment

There are many treatment options for VaIN in part because no one treatment approach gives uniform success with a single application and each approach has its unique side effect profile. Treatment depends on the age of the patient, patient's comorbidities, site of disease (i.e., near the bladder or rectum, vault after hysterectomy), multifocality, importance of preserving sexual function, risk of recurrence, physician experience and preference, and patient preference.

Table 1. Outcomes with observation alone for VaIN

Study	Include	No	Prior hyst	Technique	Median FUP	Regress	Persist	Progress Cancer	Recur
Gunderson 2013 [23]	Vain 1 Vain 2 Vain 3	26 14 4			18 mos	39% 33% 75%	54% 57% 25%		
Massad 2007 [14]	VaIN 1 VaIN 2	8 1				67%	33% 100%	0	
Ratnaelvu 2013 [24]		31				100%			
Rhodes 2014 2000-2008 [4]	VaIN 2/3	40		Intravaginal Estrogen No Estrogen		90% 71.4%			
Rome 2000 [25]	VaIN 1					88%			

Table 2. Outcomes for treatment using Trichloroacetic acid for VaIN

Study	Include	No	Prior hyst	Technique	Median FUP	Regress	Persist	Progress Cancer	Recur
Lin 2005 2001-2003 [26]	VaIN 1 VaIN 2/3	11 17		50% TCA once weekly x 4 weeks	12 mos	100% 53%			28.5%

2.1. Medical Management

The indications for topical treatment include the presence of multifocal vaginal disease and women with comorbidities that preclude an anesthetic. Medical management should not be used in women with suspected or proven invasive disease.

2.1.1. Tricholoracetic Acid

Lin [26] showed that medical management with 50% Trichloroacetic acid worked best in lower grades of VaIN. In their study of 28 women with VaIN after hysterectomy, all those with VaIN 1 went into remission compared to only 53% with VaIN 2 or 3 (OR 3.5 95% CI 1.11-11.6, p = 0.036).

2.1.2. Imiquimod (Aldara; 3M Health Care Limited, Loughborough, UK)

The concept behind imiquimod is that cytokines are known to stimulate the induction of natural killer cells which exhibit a cytotoxic action to the HPV-infected and carcinogenic cells [27]. Use of Imiquimod for VaIN is off label. Doses and schedule can range from once weekly to be scaled up to 3 times per week. Series describe self application versus direct application in the colposcopy clinic. Series show with mixed short and long term success. Series by and large involve only women with earlier grade disease. The frequency and duration of application vary across the series [27, 28]; for example, 5% cream 1-3 times per week up to 8 weeks [29]. Outcomes vary across the series and include resolution of the lesion and/or resolution of HPV.

Benefits include making a lesion smaller to allow an excisional procedure. In low grade VaIN, there is a high regression rate (86%). In high grade VaIN there is an high (85.7%) recurrence rate.

Side effects include a burning sensation, soreness and rarely, systemic effects. These side effects are not severe enough to stop treatment.

More standardized treatment protocols and longer FUP is needed to make conclusions on effectiveness and durability of treatment.

2.1.3. Topical 5Fluorouracil (5FU)

Topical 5FU is used in treating extensive or multifocal high grade VaIN. This use of 5FU is off label. The recommended doses and frequency vary from ½ applicator (1g) weekly for 6 weeks to 2g once weekly for 10-12 weeks to bid for 14-28 days [6]. After the cream is inserted usually in the evening, then half a tampon is put in the vagina and removed the next morning. Barrier cream like petroleum jelly or zinc oxide can be put on the vulva to minimize irritation. Gloves should be used when handling the medication.

Table 3. Outcomes for use of imiquimod as treatment for VaIN

Study	Include	No	Prior hyst	Technique	Median FUP	Regress	Persist	Progress Cancer	Recur
Buck 2003 [27]	VaIN 1	56 42		5% weekly x 3		86%			
Chen 2013 2006-2009 [30]	aIN 1 VaIN 2	10 2		Applicator 2x/wk x 8 wks	3mos				50%
Diakomanolis 2002 [28]	VaIN 1 VaIN 2 VaIN 3	3 2 1		5% 3x/wk For 8 wks					
Haidopoulos 2005 [31]	VaIN 2 VaIN 3	1 7			18.4mos				85.7%

Table 4. Outcomes for use of 5FU as treatment for VaIN

Study	Include	No	Prior hyst	Technique	Median FUP	Regress	Persist	Progress Cancer	Recur
Audet-LaPointe 1990 [32]		12		OD x 5 days	9-42 mos	83%			
Ballon 1979 [5]		12		2x/day x 2 weeks	6-30 mos	75%			
Caglar 1981 [33]		25		1x/d x 5-10 day	3-48 mos	85%			
Daly 1980 [34]	VaIN 2/3	17		2x/d x 10-14d	2-5 yr	100%			
Dodge 2001 [11]		22			7mos+	41%			
Gonzalez 1981 [35]		30			24 mos			1	10%
Gunderson 2013 [23]	Vain 1 Vain 2 Vain 2	1			18 mos				
Kirwan 1985 [5]		14		Weekly x 10 wk	4-42 mos	93%			
Krebs 1989 [36]		37		Weekly x 10 wk	12-84 mos	81%			
Murta 2005 [22]		16		Weekly x 10 wk	NR	62.5%			
Petrilli 1980 [5]		15		2x/d x 5-10d	2-60 mos	80%			
Piver 1979 [5]		8		1x/d x 5d/mos x 2-3 mos	3-7yr	62%			
Rome 2000 [25]	VaIN 2/3	11				46%			
Sillman 1985 [37, 38]		16							12.5%
Woodruff 1975 [5]		9			6wk-6yr	89%			

Audet [29] – 1-2 mL of 5% cream once weekly; Caglar [29] – 5 g of 5% cream applied nightly for 5 nights; Gonzalez [35] - 1.5 g once weekly for 10 wk; Woodruff [5]– 2x/day x 1mos.

Effectiveness: The effectiveness of 5FU varies across studies from 50-100%. In part the issue is the quality of the studies, and in particular details about the included population vary. In general, it is felt that the effectiveness of 5FU is lower than other therapeutic options. This may be related to poor compliance, morbidity, and VaIN that is buried and so no treated.

Benefits: The convenience of self-administration.

Side effects: These include vaginal burning, local irritation to vulva, dysparunia, ulcers, discharge and rare reports of vaginal adenosis [6]. Chronic epithelia ulcers are reported in 8% of when who used it for more than 10 weeks. When this occurs, the ulcer must be excide and closed primarily [6].

2.1.4. Poly-Y-glutamic acid (Y-PGA)

This is a naturally occurring anionic polymer produced by bacteria (Bacillus). Work in a mouse tumor model has shown antitumor activity by initiating an innate immune response.

Effectiveness: Koo [3] assessed 12 women who received this agent. There was cytologic regression in 41.7%. There was a statistically significant fall in oncogenic HPV viral load with the use of Y–PGA (p = 0.084).

Side effects: Koo [33] did not comment on side effects.

2.1.5. Cryotherapy

Although the use of cryotherapy for VaIN has been described, outcomes are poor [8] so it is not recommended.

2.1.6. Photodynamic Therapy

Photodynamic therapy involves use of light waves after exposure to a photosensitizing agent. In Choi [39], the agent was an intravenous injection of 2mg/kg photosensitizer (PSZ; Photgem R) and then 48 hr later using surface photoillumination with a 630-nm red laser light to the lesion at 150 J/cm^2. In Fehr, 10% 5-aminolevulinic acid (ALA)-gel was applied topically. After 2-4 hr, a laser light at 635 nm was applied at 80-125 J/cm^2 [40].

Effectiveness: Table 6 shows that the numbers of cases are low and the studies are mixed with patients who have VIN and/or VaIN. Regression rates are reports at 57-66%.

Benefits: The benefits of this therapy are that it preserves normal anatomy and thus, sexual function. Failures occurred in women with hyperplastic lesions or multifocal disease (OR 2.17, 95%CI 1.15-4.08, p = 0.02) [40].

Side effects: Discomfort lasts 4.9 ± 3.4 days [40].

Table 5. Outcomes of Poly-Υ-glutamic acid (Υ-PGA) as treatment for VaIN

Study	Include	No	Prior hyst	Technique	Median FUP	Regress	Persist	Progress Cancer	Recur
Koo 2015 [3]	VaIN 1 VaIN 2 VaIN 3	7 2 3			4.5mos	50%	8.3%	25%	

Table 6. Outcomes of Cryotherapy as treatment for VaIN

Study	Include	No	Prior hyst	Technique	Median FUP	Regress	Persist	Progress Cancer	Recur
Audet-LaPointe 1990 [32]	VaIN 1	1					1		
Gunderson 2013 [23]	Vain 1 Vain 2 Vain 2	1							

Table 7. Outcomes for PDT as treatment for VaIN

Study	Include	No	Prior hyst	Technique	Median FUP	Regress	Persist	Progress Cancer	Recur
Choi 2015 2003-2013 [36]	VaIN	5		PDT					
Fehr 2002 [40]	VIN/VaIN 1 VIN/VAIN 2/3	16 22		PDT		57% 66%			

2.2. Surgical Management

Surgical management requires some form of analgesia (local, spinal, epidural) or a general anaesthesia. This can be contraindicated in women with major comorbidities.

2.2.1. Laser Ablation

CO_2 laser ablation should only be considered if a biopsy shows no invasive disease and if the whole lesion can be visualized. Laser is usually performed under local or general anaesthesia. The thickness of VaIN ranges from 0.1-0.14 mm. Thus the depth to laser should be 1.5-2.0 mm [6, 41, 42]. Some suggest lasering a 5-7mm margin of normal around the lesion [43]. Perotta recommends using a 1.5mm spot diameter to depth of 1.5mm at power density of 1,130 W/ml. Watt setting of 25.4W [38]. Massad recommends laser settings of 750-1000W/mm^2 continuous beam [42]. Many physicians use topical estrogen for 1-2 weeks prior to laser ablation to allow the lesion to become more apparent.

Effectiveness: Reports vary depending on the grade, size of lesion, whether only one or more than one treatment is used, and length of follow-up. Usually a third of patients require a second treatment [6]. Cure rates are in the order of 60-90%. These cure rates are lower than laser excision. There is only one randomized trial of laser compared to CUSA. In 110 patients, there was no difference in recurrence at one year 26% versus 24% [6]. Kim showed that predictors for recurrence in 162 patients who had laser was age greater or less than 48 (OR 2.07, CI 1.18-7.01) and presence of VaIN 3 (OR 8.42, 95% CI 1.63-18.56) [44].

Benefits: Laser ablation is a versatile treatment especially of multifocal disease. It does not sacrifice vaginal epithelium and the tissues heal satisfactorily with minimal scarring (i.e., minimal sexual dysfunction).

Disadvantages: Laser requires expensive equipment and an experienced operator. It is difficult to treat buried vaginal cuff epithelium because of technical difficulties in applying laser to a folding and often distorted cuff surface within a confined space. With ablation there is the possibility of overlooking cancer.

Side effects: There is little impact on sexual and psychological function. There is minimal pain, or scarring, or risk to surrounding structures. Bleeding rates are reported at 20% [6].

2.2.2. Loop Electrosurgical Procedure (LEEP)

When using LEEP for VaIN, it is best if a wheel of local analgesic (i.e., xylocaine) is used to separate the vaginal epithelium from the underlying tissue (i.e., bladder and/or rectum depending on the location of the lesion) [6, 41]. Massad recommends a 7 x 10 mm loop with pure cutting and a 50 W ball cautery for fulguration [41]. Rather than suturing the area which can lead to scarring, it is best to leave the area open and possibly pack it for 24 hours.

Effectiveness: The number of studies and the number of patients in each study are small. The success rates are high but this technique requires more investigation.

Benefits: LEEP is a quick procedure. The power generating equipment is usually available. The loops and ball cautery may be expensive to procure. They are generally only for single use.

Complications: LEEP has the significant risk of damaging underlying structures and leading to fistula to bowel or bladder.

2.2.3. Cavitational Ultrasonic Surgical Aspiration (CUSA)

CUSA selectively removes tissue while preserving the surrounding normal tissue. Equipment can be expensive to procure and maintain.

Effectiveness: Most studies on this technique are retrospective, with only one randomized trial comparing outcomes from CUSA to Laser. In this study of 110 patients, there was no difference in recurrence rates at one year 26% versus 24% [6].

Benefits: Minimal scarring with this technique.

Side effects: Need for General Anaesthesia

2.2.4. Upper Vaginectomy

This is the preferred treatment strategy for women with VaIN 3 in the vaginal site of the hysterectomy scar. The vaginectomy can be approached vaginally, or abdominal by laparoscopy or laparotomy.

Effectiveness: This technique provides the highest success rate with 1 treatment i.e., 80-100%.

Benefits: An upper vaginectomy provides a tissue specimen to rule out cancer and assess margins [6]. Of the 105 specimens in Indermaur's study [60], there was no disease in 22% and invasive disease in 12%.

Side effects: Upper vaginectomy requires a form of anesthesia. Acute complications can include bleeding and infection. Longer term issues include vesico or recto-vaginal fistula, vaginal shortening, scarring and pain.

Table 8. Outcomes for Laser ablation as treatment for VaIN

Study	Include	No	Prior hyst	Technique	Median FUP	Regress	Persist	Progress Cancer	Recur
Audet-LaPointe 1990 [38]		32			7-85 mos	78%			
Campagnutta 1999 [5]		39			13-90 mos	33%			
Capen 1982 [5]		15			4-28 mos	80%			
Choi 2013 [45]		4				0			
Curtin 1985 [5]		27			6-42 mos	89%			
Diakomanolis 1996 [46]		25			35-82%	68%			32%
Dodge 2001 [11]		42			7mos +	63%			
Frega 2007 [47]		44	44	Laser					15/44 34% 34mos
Gunderson 2013 [23]	Vain 1	8		Laser	18 mos	73%			
	Vain 2	18			1-194 mos	61%			
	Vain 2	16				31%			
Hoffman 1991 [5]		26			11-56%	58%			5.5%
Ireland 1988 [5]		11			3-12 mos	65%			
Jobson 1983 [48]	VaIN 2/3	24			6-27mos	83% 1 tx 17% 2 tx			
Julian 1992 [5]		10			NR	70%			
Krebs 1989 [36]		22			12-84 mos	73%			
Kim 2009 1998-2007 [44]	VaIN 1	24			33mos				26.5%
	VaIN 2	18			10-115				
	VaIN 3	26							
Lenchan 1986 [5]		22			6-27 mos	50%			
Massad 2007 [42]	VaIN 2	3				2 (67%)	1(33%)		
	VaIN 3	6				5 (83%)	1(17%)		

Table 8. (Continued)

Study	Include	No	Prior hyst	Technique	Median FUP	Regress	Persist	Progress Cancer	Recur
Omer 2003 [49]	VaIN 2/3	24				70.8% with 1 tx 79.2% with multiple			33%
Perrotta 2013 2003-2009 [43]	VaIN 2/3	21			25mos 12-78mos	86%	10%		4%
Petrelli 1980 [5]		10			2-12mos	90%			
Ramirez 2015 [50]									
Rome 2000 [25]	Vain 2/3	26				69%			
Stafle 1977 [5]		8			3-12	87%			
Stuart 1988 [5]		22			6-38 mos	85%			
Supracordevole 1998 [5]		24			3-12mos	67%			
Townsend 1982 [5]		36			NR	78%			
Von Gruenigen 2007 [51]	VaIN 1 VaIN 2/3	16 11							15.4%
Wang 2014 [52]	VaIN 1 VaIN 2 VaIN 3	20 10 9 39				15 (75%) 3 (30%)	3 (15%) 7 (70%) 9 (100%)		2 (10%)
Woodman 1984 [53]		14			6-60mos	43%			
Yalcin 1990-1998 [54]	VaIN 2/3	33				70.8% with 1 79.2% with multiple		1/33 (3%)	

Table 9. Outcomes of using LEEP as treatment for VaIN

Study	Include	No.	Prior hyst	Technique	Median FUP	Regress	Persist	Progress Cancer	Recur
Fanning 1999 [38]		15							
Massad 2007 [42]	VaIN 1	4				100%			
Terzakis 2010 [55]		23			12 mos 24 mos	86.96% 75%			13.04% 25%
Terzakis 2011 [556]		8	Prior history of cervical cancer	80 watt	12 mos 24 mos	75% 62.5%			25% 37.5%

Table 10. Outcomes of CUSA as treatment for VaIN

Study	Include	No	Prior hyst	Technique	Median FUP	Regress	Persist	Progress Cancer	Recur
Matsuo 2009 [57]		92			4.5 yr			0	20%
Robinson 2000 [58]	VaIN 1-3	29			33 mos	74%		0	34%
Von Gruenigen 2007 [51}	VaIN 1 VaIN 2/3	12 13							15.4%

Table 11. Outcomes of upper vaginectomy as treatment for VaIN

Study	Include	No.	Prior hyst	Technique	Median FUP	Regress	Persist	Progress Cancer	Recur
Curtis 1992 [59]		12			55 mos 9-99 mos	83%		8.3%	
Diakomanolis 2002 [38]		24							21%
Dodge 2001 [11]		13			7 mos	100%			
Gunderson 2013 [23]	Vain 1 Vain 2 Vain 2	13			18 mos				
Hoffman 1992 [5, 38]		32			19.5 mos 6-73 mos	83%			17%
Indermaur 2005 1985-2004 [60]	VaIN 2/3	105			25 mos	88%		12% in specimen	6%
Lee 1976 [61]		66						1.5%	

Table12. Outcomes of local surgical excision as treatment for VaIN

Study	Include	No	Prior hyst	Technique	Median FUP	Regress	Persist	Progress Cancer	Recur
Audet-LaPointe 1990 [32]	VaIN 3	2			16-118 mos	100%			
Cheng 1999 [62]	VaIN 3	35			44 mos 1-124 mos	66%		10%	14%
Gunderson 2013 [23]	Vain 1 Vain 2 Vain 2	13 7 24			18 mos 1-194 mos	 25% 29%			
Rome 2000 [25]	VaIN 2/3	77				69%			
Woodman 1984 [53]		4			7mos-6yr	50%			

Table 13. Outcomes for total vaginectomy as treatment for VaIN

Study	Include	No	Prior hyst	Technique	Median FUP	Regress	Persist	Progress Cancer	Recur
Audet-LaPointe 1990 [32]	VaIN 3	1			76	100%			
Haidopoulos 2005 [31]		2		Vaginectomy					
Luyten 2015 2003-2013 [7]		33		Vaginectomy by laser		87% of the 23			
Laser colpectomy									
Luyten 2014 2003-2013 [7]	VaIN 2/3 lesions >20cm^2 VaIN 2 VaIN 3	23 4 19		Laser skinning vaginectomy	12 mos 12-104 mos	87%		8.6%	

Table 14. Outcomes of brachytherapy as treatment of VaIN

Study	Include	No.	Prior hyst	Technique	Median FUP	Regress	Persist	Progress Cancer	Recur
Blanchard 2011 [63]	VaIN 3	28	24	LDR 60Gy	41 mos	93%			1 3.5%
Graham 2007 [65]	VaIN 3	22		48 Gy in 2 insertions one week apart	77 mos	86.4%		2	3 14%
MacCleod 1997 [66]	VaIN 3	14		17-18 Gy per week x 3 wk 42.5 Gy in 8.5 Gy per fraction to a depth of 0.5-1.0 cm at the vault	46 mos	12 85.7%	1	1	7%
Ogino 1998 [64]	VaIN 3	6		HDR 23.3Gy 25-30 Gy in 5 Gy per fraction to depth of 1.0 cm at apex	90mos	100%			0
Rome 2015 [25]	VaIN 2/3	2				2 (100%)			
Song 2014 1998-2011 [17]	VaIN 1 VaIN 2 VaIN 3 ?	34 6 6 1 9	34	40Gy in 8 fractions over 4 weeks HDR-ICR Iridium 192 source	48mos 4-122 mos	88.2%	2		2
Woodman 1988 [53]		11	11	LDR 27-51 Gy	25mos	12	100%		

2.2.5. Surgical Excision

Surgically removing a lesion can be facilitated by using local analgesia with or without adrenaline to lift the vagina off underlying tissues so as to prevent trauma to surrounding areas. Goal is to remove 5mm of normal epithelium around the lesion [29].

Effectiveness: Success rates are 25-69%.

Side effects: Upper vaginectomy requires a general or spinal/epidural anesthetic. Acute complications can include bleeding and infection. Longer term issues include vescico or rectal fistula, vaginal shortening, scarring and pain.

2.2.6. Total Vaginectomy

A total vaginectomy can be accomplished using either a vaginal or abdominal approach. There is the opportunity to use split thickness skin grafts or flaps to reconstruct the vagina.

This is not the best strategy for those women who are interested in preserving the ability to have sexual activity. Luyten [7] described using CO_2 laser to complete the total vaginectomy. In his report, the patients were heavily pretreated and 10 had cancer in the specimen.

Benefits: Total vaginectomy has the lowest recurrence rates of 12% [6]

Side effects: These include vesico-vaginal fistula, recto-vaginal fistula, and skin graft necrosis. Recurrences have been reported in skin grafts used to create a neovagina [6].

2.3. Brachytherapy

Brachytherapy is usually used when VaIN cases are resistant to conventional medical and/or surgical treatment. Brachytherapy is usually used in women who are poor surgical candidates or if there is multifocal disease.

Outcomes: There are six studies describing the use of vaginal brachytherapy for treating VaIN. It is a mixed group of technologies including low dose rate [63] and high dose rate [17, 64]. Various radiation techniques were used across the studies (ie. ovoids versus vaginal cylinder) [17]. Many of the women had had a prior hysterectomy. By and large, the women had VaIN 3 and they had failed other types of treatment [23]. Disease regression rates were high, persistence low, progression to cancer low [65, 66], and recurrence rates low [17, 65].

Side effects: Higher doses per fraction are usually associated with more late normal tissue toxicity [17].

Although the authors report a low rate of grade 3-4 toxicities, radiation is not usually a front line treatment. Premature ovarian failure can occur in young women. Vaginal atrophy can occur [32]. The vagina scarring with or without stenosis and vaginal shortening does compromise sexual function and satisfaction (Graham [65] reported 3/22 cases of grade 3 vaginal stenosis) (Song [16] reported 3/34 vaginal stricture with dysparunia). This can make follow-up difficult. There can be rectal bleeding especially with high radiation doses.

There is a risk of developing cancer. Once a person receives vaginal brachytherapy, conservative treatment is no longer an option due to the damage that radiation has on blood vessels and connective tissue. If surgery is used after radiation there is a difficulty with poor healing.

Risk for Recurrence after Treatment

A few authors have tried to understand the reasons for recurrence and the relative importance of these reasons compared to others. Dodge assessed the reasons for recurrence. He showed that the most important reason was the method of treatment (OR 22.4, 95% CI 1.3-393.6, p = 0.001) (5FU had higher rate of recurrence then laser) and multifocal disease also was important (OR 3.3 95%CI 1.2-9.2, p = 0.02) [11]. Matsuo suggested that high grade VaIN had a 32.3% risk of recurrence compared to low grade VaIN 1.31%, (p = 0.044) [57].

Limitations of Studies

The studies listed in the Tables above are by and large, retrospective nature. This introduces selection bias. The stringency of the inclusion and exclusion criteria is clearly outlined in Gunderson [23]; but many of the other studies include women with VaIN 1 with VaIN 2-3, first treatment versus multiple treatments, presence of synchronous primaries (vulva and/or cervix with VaIN). The recruitment period is often long. There is lack of detail on lesion size. The outcome variables are often not clearly defined. The studies may or may not report the duration of follow-up or the follow-up strategy and these may have changed over time. They may or may not report the lost to follow-up rate. In part these issues are related to the small number of women with this disease and the lack of centralization of their care.

Strategy

There are some themes that have been gleaned over time.

Firstly, when selecting a treatment it is important to consider prior treatment, whether the disease is multifocality, patient's other comorbidities, and the woman's desire to preserve sexual function. For example, in a young woman or a woman with multifocal disease, laser or medical management is the first line of treatment.

A second principal is that VaIN 1 (condyloma) often regresses spontaneously and it does not have a malignant potential. Thus, close surveillance without treatment is preferable. Follow-up is recommended as it does tend to recur frequently [4]. If treatment is used try topical intravaginal application of estrogen [7]. Conservative management is an option for majority of VaIN 2 and selected VaIN 3.

A third principal is that surgical management like excision or ablation (laser, LEEP or CUSA) all require that the lesion is fully visible and has been adequately biopsied to exclude invasive disease.

A forth principal is that multifocal VaIN 2/3 needs a versatile approach like medical management or laser.

A fifth principal is that an upper vaginectomy the treatment of choice for post-hysterectomy vaginal apex VaIN 3.

A sixth principal is that radical options like brachytherapy or total vaginectomy should be reserved for highly selected cases like those women who have had multiple recurrences, or multifocal disease.

FOLLOW-UP

Although some women are successfully treated with their first strategy, follow-up is recommended as a third of women require a second treatment. Stillman [8] reported on 74 women. 70% went into remission with one treatment and 94% with a second treatment. Some of the reasons for treatment failure in this group included the presence of multifocal lesions, and anogenital neoplastic syndrome (i.e., dysplasia in more than one lower genital tract site). However, in this group factors that were not involved in treatment failure included: VaIN grade, associated cervical neoplasia and immunosuppression.

There is no optimal follow-up strategy. Some suggest vaginal cytology every 6 months for 2 years and then annually. Ratnavelu [24] showed that if the cytology was high grade after treatment then 79% developed recurrence at a median of 7 months (Range 2-21 months) (HR 5.6 95% 2.0-15.5, p = 0.001). There may be a role for HPV testing but this is not yet define [6]. The role of colposcopic follow-up with or instead of cytology is not clear. In addition to follow-up with cytology, women should be counseled to stop smoking

PRIMARY PREVENTION

In a chapter on VaIN, we would be remiss not to point out the incredible value of primary prevention. This chapter has shown the difficulty of living with VaIN and the poor outcomes after treatment, need for repeated treatments and risk for malignancy. Given that 64% of VaIN 2-3 is related to oncogenic HPV, there is the potential to prevent this disease through vaccination [67]. Some reports suggest close to 100% efficacy of vaccine in preventing disease if vaccinated prior to infection. The benefits of pre-exposure vaccination with the nanovalent HPV vaccine are so evident in preventing CIN, VaIN, VIN, PaIN and cancers related to these sites [67].

REFERENCES

[1]   Alemany L, Saunier M, Inoco L, Quiros B, Alvarado-Cabrero I, Alejo M, Joura EA et al. Large contribution of human papillomavirus in vaginal neoplastic lesions: a worldwide study in 597 samples. *Eur J Cancer* 2014;50(16):2846-54.

[2]   American Cancer Society's (ACS) publication, Cancer Facts & Figures 2015, and the ACS website. Accessed August 31, 2015.

[3]   Koo YJ, Min KJ, Hong JH, Lee JK. Efficacy of poly-gamma-glutamic acid in women with high-risk human papillomavirus-positive vaginal intraepithelial Neoplasia: an observational pilot study. *J Microbiol Biotechnol* 2015.

[4]   Rhodes HE, Chenevert L, Munsell M. Vaginal Intraepithelial Neoplasia (VaIN 2/3): comparing clinical outcomes of treatment with intravaginal estrogen. *JLGTD* 2014:18(2):115-121.

[5]   Holschneider CH, Berek JS. Vaginal intraepithelial Neoplasia. 2015 UpToDate® Pages 1-14.

[6]   Gurumurthy M, Cruickshank ME. Management of vaginal intraepithelial Neoplasia. *JLTGD* 2012;16(3):306-12.

[7]   Luyten A, Hastor H, Vasileva T, Zander M, Petry KU. Laser-skinning colpectomy for extended vaginal intraepithelial Neoplasia and microinvasive cancer. *Gynecol Onc* 2014:135(2):217-222.

[8]   Cardosi RJ. Bomalaski JJ, Hoffman MS. Diagnosis and management of vulvar and vaginal intraepithelial Neoplasia. *Obstet Gynecol Clin North Am* 2001;28(4):685-702.

[9]   Aho M, Vesterinen E, Meyer B et al: Natural history of vaginal intraepithelial neoplasia. *Cancer* 1991:68;195-197.

[10]   Bornstein J, Kaufman RH: Combination of surgical excision and carbon dioxide laser vaporization for multifocal vulvar intraepithelial neoplasia. *Am J Obstet Gynecol* 1988;158:459-464.

[11]   Dodge JA, Eltabbakh GH, Mount SL, Walder RP, Morgan A. Clinical features and risk of recurrence among patients with vaginal intraepithelial Neoplasia. *Gynecol Oncol* 2001;83(2):363-9.

[12]   Boonlikit S, Noinual N. Vaginal intraepithelial neoplasia: a retrospective analysis of clinical features and colpohistology. *J Obstet Gynecol Res* 2010;36(1):94-100.

[13]   Sherman JF, Mount SL, Evans MF, Skelly J, Simmons-Arnold L, Eltabbakh GH. Smoking increases the risk of high-grade vaginal intraepithclial Neoplasia in women with oncogenic human papillomavirus. *Gyn Oncol* 2008;110(3):396-401.

[14]   Massad LS, Xie X, Greenblatt RM, Minkoff H, Sanchez-Keeland L, Watts DH, Wright RL, D'Souza G, Merenstein D, Strickler H. Effect of human immunodeficiency virus infection on the prevalence and incidence of vaginal intraepithelial Neoplasia. *Obstet Gynecol* 2012;119(3):582-9.

[15]   Chao A, Chen TC, Hsueh C, Huang CC, Yang JE, Hsueh S, Huang HJ, Lin CT, Tang YH, Liou JD, Chang CJ, Chou HH, Lai CH. Human papillomavirus in vaginal intraepithelial Neoplasia. *Int J Cancer* 2012; 131(3):E259-68.

[16]   Schockaert S, Poppe W, Arbyn M, Verguts T, Vergut J. Incidence of vaginal intraepithelial after hysterectomy for cervical intraepithelial Neoplasia: a retrospective study. *Am J Obstet Gynecol* 2008;199 (2):113.

[17]   Song JH, Lee JH, Lee JH, Park JS, Hong SH, Jang HS, Kim YS, Choi BO, Yoon SC. High-dose rate brachytherapy for treatment of vaginal intraepithelial Neoplasia. *Cancer Res Treat* 2014;46(1):74-80.

[18] Li Z, Barron S, Hong W, Karunamurthy A, Zhao C. Surveillance for recurrent cancers and vaginal epithelial lesions in patients with invasive cervical cancer after hysterectomy: are vaginal cytology and high-risk human papillomavirus testing useful? *Am J Clin Pathol* 2013;140(5):708-14.

[19] Li H, Guo YL, Zhang JX, Qiao J, Geng L. Risk factors for the development of vaginal intraepithelial Neoplasia. *Chin Med J* 2012;125(7):1219-23.

[20] So KA, Hong JH, Hwang JH, Song SH, Lee JK, Lee NW, Lee KW. The utility of the human papillomavirus DNA load for the diagnosis and prediction of persistent vaginal intraepithelial neoplasia. *J Gynecol Oncol* 2009;20(4):232-7.

[21] Cheung KW, Cheung VY. Hysterectomy for abnormal cervical smear when local excision is not possible. *JLTGD* 2014;18(3):235-9.

[22] Murta EF, Neves Junior MA, Sempionato LR, Costa MC, Maluf PJ. Vaginal intraepithelial neoplasia: clinical therapeutic analysis of 33 cases. *Arch Gynecol Obstet* 2005;272(4):261-4.

[23] Gunderson CC, Nugent EK, Elfrink SH, Gold MA, Moore KN. A contemporary analysis of epidemiology and management of vaginal intraepithelial Neoplasia. *Am J Obstet Gynecol* 2013;208(5):410 e1-6.

[24] Ratnavelu N, Patel A, Fisher AD, Galaal K, Cross P, Naik R. High-grade vaginal intraepithelial Neoplasia: can we be selective about who we treat? *BJOG* 2013;20(7):887-93.

[25] Rome RM, England PG. Management of vaginal intraepithelial Neoplasia: a series of 132 cases with long-term follow-up. Int J Gynecol *Cancer.* 2000;10(5):382-390.

[26] Lin H, Huang EY, Chang HY, ChangChien CC. Therapeutic effect of topical applications of trichloroacetic acid for vaginal intraepithelial neoplasia after hysterectomy. *Jpn J Clin Oncol* 2005;35(11):651-4.

[27] Buch HW, Guth KJ. Treatment of vaginal intraepithelial neoplasia (primarily low grade) with imiquimod 5% cream. JLGTD 2003;7(4):290-3.

[28] Diakomanolis E, Haidopoulos D, Stafanidis K. Treatment of High-grade vaginal intraepithelial Neoplasia with imiquimod cream. *N Engl J Med* 2002;347(5):374.

[29] Nelson EL, Stockdale CK. Vulvar and Vaginal HPV Disease. *Obstet Gynecol Clin N Am* 2013;40:359-376.

[30] Chen FP. Efficacy of imiquimod 5% cream for persistent human papillomavirus in genital intraepithelial neoplasm. *Taiwan J Obstet Gynecol* 2013;52(4):475-8.

[31] Haidopoulos D, Diakomanolis E, Rodolakis A, Voulgaris Z, Vlachos G, Intsaklis A. Can local application of imiquimod cream be an alternative mode of therapy for patients with high grade intraepithelial lesions of the vagina? *Int J Gynecol Cancer* 2005;15(5):898-902.

[32] Audet-LaPointe P, Body C, Vauclair R, Drouin P, Ayoub J. Vaginal Intraepithelial neoplasia. *Gynecol Oncol* 1990;36:232-239.

[33] Caglar H, Hertzog RW, Hreshchyshyn MM. Topical 5-fluorouracil treatment of vaginal intraepithelial Neoplasia. *Obstet Gynecol* 1981;58:580-3.

[34] Daly JW, Ellis GF. Treatment of vaginal dysplasia and carcinoma in situ with topical 5-fluorouracil. *Obstet Gynecol* 1980;55:350-2.

[35] Gonzalez Sanchez JL, Flores Murrieta G, Chavez Brambila J, Deolarte Manzano JM, Andard Manzan AF. Topical 5-flurouracil for treatment of vaginal intraepithelial neoplasms (in Spanish). *Ginecol Obstet Mex* 2002;70:244-7.

[36] Krebs HB. Treatment of vaginal intraepithelial neoplasia with laser and topical 5-fluorouracil. *Obstet Gynecol* 1989;73:657-60.

[37] Sillman FH, Sedlis A, Boyce J. 5-FU/chemosurgery for difficult lower genital intraepithelial neoplasia. *Contemp Obstet Gynecol* 1985;27:79-101.

[38] Frega A, Sopracordevole F, Assorgi C, Lombardi D, EC Sanctis V, Catalano A, Matteuci E, Milazzo GN, Ricciardi E, Moscarini M. Vaginal intraepithelial Neoplasia: a therapeutical dilemma. *Anticancer Res* 2013;33(1):29-38.

[39] Choi MC, Kim MS, Lee GH, Jung SG, Park H, Joo WD, Lee C, Lee JH, Hwang YY, Kim SJ. Photodynamic therapy for premalignant lesions of the vulva and vagina: a long term follow-up study. *Lasers Surg Med* 2015 14.

[40] Fehr MK, Hornung R, Degen A, Schwarz VA, Fink D, Haller U, Wyss P. Photodynamic therapy of vulvar and vaginal condyloma and intraepithelial Neoplasia using topically applied 5-aminolevulinic acid. *Lasers Surg Med* 2002;30(4):273-9.

[41] Benedet JL, Vilson PS, Matisic JP: Epidermal thickness measurements in vaginal intraepithelial neoplasia: A basis for optimal CO2 laser vaporization. *J Reprod Med* 1992;37:809-812.

[42] Massad LS. Outcomes after diagnosis of vaginal intraepithelial Neoplasia. *JLTGD* 2007;16-19.

[43] Perrotta M, Marchitelli CE, Velazco AF, Tauscher P, Lopez G, Peremateu MS. Use of CI2 laser vaporization for the treatment of high-grade vaginal intraepithelial Neoplasia. *JLTGD* 2013:17(1):23-7.

[44] Kim HS, Park NH, Park IA, Park JH, Chung HH, Kim JW, Song YS, Kang SB. Risk factors for recurrence of vaginal intraepithelial Neoplasia in the vaginal vault after laser vaporization. *Lasers Surg Med.* 2009;41(3):196-202.

[45] Choi YJ, Hur SY, Park JS, Lee KH. Laparoscopic upper vaginectomy for post-hysterectomy high risk vaginal intraepithelial Neoplasia and syperficially invasive vaginal carcinoma. *World J Surg Oncol* 2013:11:126.

[46] Diakomanolis E,Rodolakis A, Boulgaris Z, Blachos G, Michalas S. Treatment of vaginal intraepithelial neoplasia with laser ablation and upper Vaginectomy. *Gynecol Obstet* 2002;54(1):17-20.

[47] Frega A, French D, Piazze J, Cerekja A, Vetrano G, Moscarini M. Prediction of persistent vaginal intraepithelial neoplasia in previously hysterectomized women by high-risk HPV DNA detection. *Cancer Lett* 2007;249(2):235-41.

[48] Jobson VW, Homesley HD. Treatment of vaginal intraepithelial neoplasia with the carbon dioxide laser. *Obstet Gynecol* 1983;62:90-3.

[49] Omer TY, Rutherford TJ, Chambers SK, Chambers JT, Schwartz PE. Vaginal intraepithelial neoplasia: treatment by carbon dioxide laser and reisk factors for failure. *Eur J Obstet Gynecol Reprod Biol* 2003;106:64-8.

[50] Ramirez S, Barrena N, Conell YM, Torres P, Leon H, Jimenez P, Acuna D, Meneses M. Laser vaporization in Vulvar Intraepithelial Neoplasia (VIN), Vaginal intraepithelial neoplasia (VAIN) and condylomata acuminate: IGCS-0093 Vular and Vaginal Cancer. *Int J Gynecol Cancer* 2015:Supp 1:75.

[51] Von Gruenigen VE, Gibbons HE, Gibbins K, Jenison EL, Hopkins MP. Surgical treatments for vulvar and vaginal dysplasia: a randomized controlled trial. *Obstet Gynecol* 2007;109(4):942-7.

[52] Wang Y, Kong WM, Wu YM, Wang JD, Zhang WY. Therapeutic effect of laser vaporization for vaginal intraepithelial Neoplasia following hysterectomy due to premalignant and malignant lesions. *J Obstet Gynecol Res.* 2014;40(6):1740-7.

[53] Woodman CB, Mould JJ, Jordan JA. Radiotherapy in the management of vaginal intraepithelial neoplasia after hysterectomy. *Br J Obstet Gynecol* 1988;95:976-9.

[54] Yalcin OT, Rutherford TJ, Chambers SK, Chambers JT, Schwartz PE. Vaginal intraepithelial neoplasia: treatment by carbon dioxide laser and risk factors for failure. *Eur J Obstet Gynecol Reprod Biol* 2003;106(1):64-9.

[55] Terakis E, Androutsopoulos G, Zygouris D, Grigoriadis C, Arnogiannaki N. Loop electrosurgical excision procedure In Greek patients with vaginal intraepithelial neoplasia. *Eur J Gynecol Oncol* 2010;31(4): 392-4.

[56] Terakis E, Androutsopoulos G, Zygouris D, Grigoriadis C, Arnogiannaki N. Loop electrosurgical excision procedure In Greek patients with vaginal intraepithelial neoplasia and history of cervical cancer. *Eur J Gynecol Oncol* 2011;32(5):530-3.

[57] Matsuo K, Chi DS, Walker LD, Rosenshein NB, Im DD. Ultrasonic surgical aspiration for vaginal intraepithelial Neoplasia. *Int J Gynecol Obstet* 2009;105(1):71-3.

[58] Robinson JB, Sun CC, Bodurka-Bevers D, Im DD, Rosenshein NB. Cavitational ultrasonic surgical aspiration for the treatment of vaginal intraepithelial Neoplasia. *Gynecol Oncol* 2000;78(2):235-41.

[59] Curtis P, Shepherd JH, Lowe DG et al. The role of partial colpectomy in the management of persistent vaginal neoplasia after primary treatment. *Br J Obstet Gynecol* 1992;99:587-589.

[60] Indermaur MD, Martino MA, Fiorica JV, Roberts WS, Hoffman MS. Upper vaginectomy for the treatment of vaginal intraepithelial neoplasia. *Am J Obstet Gynecol* 2005;193(2):577-80.

[61] Lee RA, Symmonds RE. Recurrent carcinoma in situ of the vagina in patients previously treated for in situ carcinoma of the cervix. Obstet Gynecol 1976;48:61-64.

[62] Cheng D, Ng TY, Ngan HYS, Wong LC. Wide local excision (WLE) for vaginal intraepithelial neoplasia (VaIN). *Acta Obstet Gynecol Scand.* 1999;78:648-52.

[63] Blanchard P, Monnier L, Dumas I, Morice P, Pautier P, Duvillard P, Azoury F, Mazeron R, Haie-Meder C. Low-dose-rate definitive brachytherapy for high-grade vaginal intraepithelial neoplasia. *Oncologist* 2011;16(2):182-8.

[64] Ogino I, Kitamura T, Okajima H, Matsubara S. High dose rate intracavitary brachytherapy in the management of cervical and vaginal intraepithelial neoplasia. *Int J Radiat Oncol Biol Phys* 1998;40:881-7.

[65] Graham K, Wright K, Cadwallader B, Reed NS, Symonds RP. 20-year retrospective review of medium dose rate intracavitary brachytherapy in VAIN 3. *Gynecol Oncol* 2007 106(1):105-111.

[66] MacCleod C, Fowler A, Dlarymple C, Atkinson K, Elliott P, Carter J. High-dose rate brachytherapy in the management of high-grade intraepithelial neoplasia of the vagina. *Gynecol Oncol* 1997:65:74-7.

[67] Joura EA, Giulano AR, Iversen DE, Boudard C, Mao C et al. for the Board Spectrum HPV Vaccine Study. A 9-valent HPV Vaccine against infection and intra epithelial neoplasia of women. *NEJM* 2015;372(8):711-23.

In: Cryosurgery and Colposcopy
Editor: Lillian Watson

ISBN: 978-1-63484-507-6
© 2016 Nova Science Publishers, Inc.

Chapter 5

VAGINAL VAULT CYTOLOGY AFTER HYSTERECTOMY

Antonios Anagnostopoulos[1,*], Bridget De Cruze[2], John Kirwan[2] and Jonathan Herod[2]
[1]Senior Registrar in Obstetrics and Gynaecology,
Liverpool Women's Hospital NHS Trust, Liverpool, UK
[2]Consultant Gynaecological Oncologists Liverpool Women's Hospital,
Liverpool, UK

ABSTRACT

Cervical dysplasia diagnosed at or before hysterectomy or recent dyskaryosis on a cervical smear are considered risk factors for the development of vaginal intraepithelial neoplasia (VaIN) following hysterectomy. Current guidance recommends vault cytology in women who are at increased risk of VaIN but evidence of benefit is weak. This is a retrospective cohort study of 330 women who had a hysterectomy for benign pathology. The follow up practice and the results of vaginal pathology were recorded 24 and 60 months following surgery. One case of high grade vaginal intraepithelial neoplasia was recorded but no cases of vaginal cancer were diagnosed in the high risk group of patients within a 5 year period post hysterectomy. Relevant studies predate routine human papilloma virus (HPV) testing and there is limited data regarding the course of vaginal HPV infections in the absence of a cervix. The

---

[*] E-mail: a.anagnostopoulos@nhs.net, phone: +44(0)7896613039.

available evidence is reviewed and an approach for the follow up of this group of women is suggested.

INTRODUCTION

Vaginal cancer is the rarest of gynaecological cancers, with approximately 260 cases diagnosed annually in the UK [1]. The most significant risk factors for its development are vaginal Intraepithelial neoplasia (VaIN), cervical intraepithelial neoplasia (CIN), or anogenital cancer [2]. Up to 80% of vaginal cancers are secondary involvement by tumours from the cervix or vulva. High grade VaIN can progress to invasion despite treatment in up to 3% of cases [3]. Despite a prolonged duration of a detectable precursor lesion; the extremely low incidence of primary vaginal cancer limits the applicability of screening. The management of women with a current or recent history of CIN or dyskaryosis who undergo hysterectomy should remain under the operating surgeon. For this group of women UK's national cervical screening programme suggests vaginal vault cytology at 6 and 18 months following hysterectomy [8]. For the same group of women the American College of Obstetricians and Gynecologists suggests 3 yearly vaginal vault cytology for up to 20 years [9]. The absence of applicable evidence leads to variation in this area of practice. Usually vaginal vault cytology is managed outside the centralised cervical screening programme and is individualised.

We therefore assessed the follow up approaches of gynaecological surgeons in a tertiary unit. Since the reported evidence predates the use of liquid based cytology (LBC), and high risk-HPV testing, we considered an alternative approach.

MATERIALS AND METHODS

All women who had undergone a total hysterectomy for an indication other than cancer, at Liverpool Women's Hospital between 1st of January 2008 and 31st of December 2008, were identified from the hospital episodes statistics database. Histology and cytology results were retrieved via the pathology and cytology electronic databases. Patients with malignancy were excluded. The presence of CIN in the hysterectomy specimen was recorded. Recent cervical cytology status of patients was recorded by accessing the nationwide electronic register for cervical screening. Follow up results for all patients were electronically sought at 30 months following hysterectomy. For patients with risk factors for VaIN (i.e *those with CIN at the hysterectomy specimen or a recent history of dyskaryosis or CIN prior to hysterectomy*), a further search was performed at 60 months following hysterectomy.

RESULTS

330 patients had undergone total hysterectomy without any histological evidence of malignancy. Previous cervical screening history could be confirmed in 292 and was normal in 211 women. Considering the risk factors mentioned above, 81 women (27.7%) were found to be at high risk for VaIN. A complete data set was available for 57 out of these 81 women. Of the remaining 57 women, 7 had cervical dysplasia in the hysterectomy specimen and 50 had a recent history of dyskaryosis or CIN (Figure 1). Within the first 30 months after surgery gynaecologists requested follow up with vaginal cytology for only 9 out of these 57 patients (15.7%). It appears that clinicians decided to follow up:

- 5 out of 7 patients (71.4%), with CIN or CGIN in the hysterectomy specimen (including one patient with incompletely excised VaIN3)
- 4 out of the 50 patients (8%), with a recent history of CIN or dyskaryosis. (3 out of these 4 patients had a previous history of high grade dysplasia treated with conisation)

The one case of VaIN3 identified during follow up was a patient with a recent history of CIN2/3 treated with conisation. This patient had a severely dyskaryotic smear at 27 months following hysterectomy. In this cohort the estimated incidence VaIN2/3 in first 2 years following hysterectomy was 0.37%. At 5 years after hysterectomy, none of the 57 high risk patients had evidence of vaginal preinvasive or invasive disease.

DISCUSSION

Using CIN at the hysterectomy specimen or a recent history of dyskaryosis or CIN prior to hysterectomy as risk factors for VaIN, approximately 25% of patients will qualify for vaginal vault cytology following a hysterectomy for benign pathology.

Clinicians mainly chose to follow up patients with dysplastic cervical lesions diagnosed at the hysterectomy. The incidence of VaIN3 following hysterectomy for reasons other than cancer in this cohort was 0.37%.

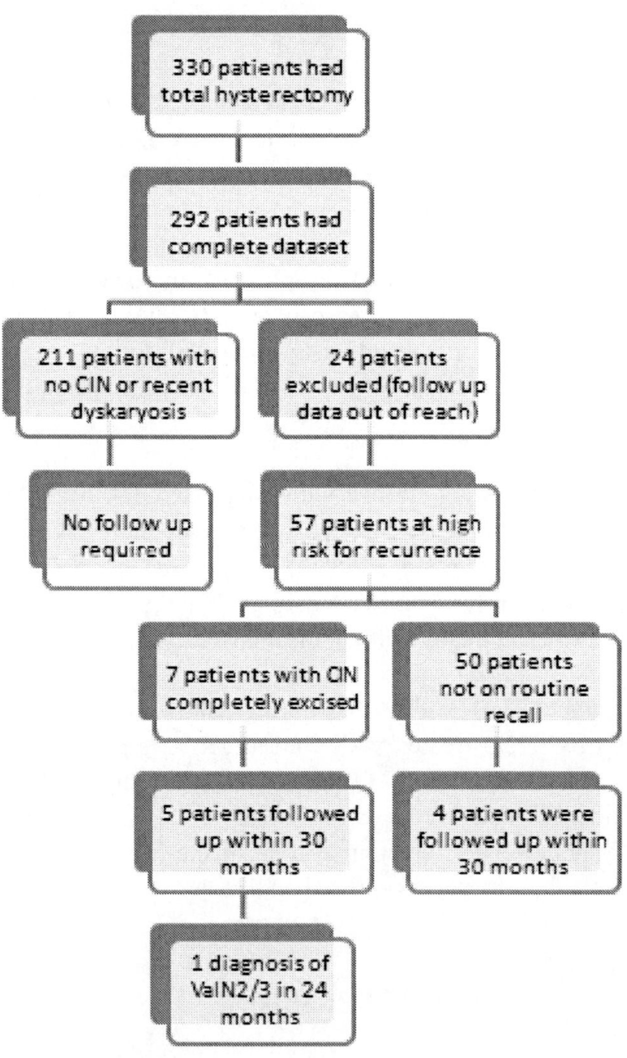

Figure 1. Follow up results.

There is conflicting evidence in literature with respect to estimating the risk of VaIN and vaginal cancer following hysterectomy in women with present or recent history of CIN2/3. A systematic review by Soutter in 2006 suggested that the risk of cancer following treatment for CIN is similar whether treatment was by cervical conisation or hysterectomy. In this review the risk of pre-invasive or invasive disease did not appear to decline earlier than 8 years following treatment [4]. A systematic review in 2006 reported only one vaginal cancer occurring after 11659 hysterectomies performed for reasons other than malignancy [5]. In 5037 of these hysterectomies CIN3 was present. However, the weakness of this review was that length of follow-up was either unknown or of less than 1 year duration in the majority of the studies included.

A more recent retrospective study of 8457 unselected vaginal vault cytology results revealed mild or moderate dyskaryosis in 4.5%, severe dyskaryosis in 1.2% and malignancy in less than 0.1% of the cases. The authors therefore questioned the cost effectiveness of follow up with vault cytology [6]. In 2014, a 50 year long cohort study including the entire Swedish population concluded that women previously treated for CIN3 are at increased risk of developing vaginal cancer at an old age [7]. Women treated before 1970 were hysterectomy was the main treatment had increased risk for development of vaginal cancer but this risk was lower compared to the ones treated later mainly with conisation.

A study adequately powered to reveal differences in the detection rate of VaIN2/3 between different follow up strategies would require an extremely large sample size. The low incidence of VaIN 2/3 [5], the prolonged follow up of 5 to 8 years along with the high drop-out rate expected, limit the feasibility of such study.

Women without CIN or CGIN in the hysterectomy specimen histopathology report and normal cervical cytology testing prior to hysterectomy should not require follow up since the risk for malignancy in this group seems negligible.

Women with current or recent history of CIN2/3, dyskaryosis or HR-HPV infection that have hysterectomy have a low but not negligible risk of VaIN2/3. We suggest these women to be recalled at 12 months for a vaginal vault LBC sample, by a colposcopy practitioner in secondary care. This appears safe since evidence does not support progression of VaIN to invasion in less than 12 months [11]. For this group primary HR-HPV testing can be initially performed. In cervical cancer studies HR-HPV test has shown a high negative predictive value for a period of 5 years [12]. Although relevant data for HR-HPV test in VaIN are lacking, studies report more than 70% presence of HR-HPV in VaIN [13]. If genital tract is clear of carcinogenic HPV serotypes following a hysterectomy women could stop further routine cytology.

In those women with positive HR-HPV test cytology should be performed and those with dyskaryosis should be referred for vaginoscopy by a gynaecologist specialised in colposcopy. If biopsies of suspected lesions confirm VaIN2/3 or invasion; women should be referred to tertiary centres for further management. Women found positive for HR-HPV which have mild or no dyskaryosis or VaIN1 can be followed up with vaginal vault LBC in 3 years' time. Immunocompromised patients should have individualised plans of care.

REFERENCES

[1]   http://www.cancerresearchuk.org/cancer-help/type/vaginal-cancer/ about/. (accessed 26 June 2014).

[2]   Sillman F. H., Fruchter R. G., Chen Y. S., Camilien L., Sedlis A., McTigue E. Vaginal intraepithelial neoplasia: risk factors for persistence, recurrence, and invasion and its management. *Am. J Obstet. Gynecol.*, 1997 Jan.; 176:93-9.

[3]   Ratnavelu N., Patel A., Fisher A. D., Galaal K., Cross P., Naik R. High-grade vaginal intraepithelial neoplasia: can we be selective about who we treat? *BJOG,* 2013 Jun.; 120(7):887-93.

[4]   Soutter W. P., Sasieni P., Panoskaltsis T. Long-term risk of invasive cervical cancer after treatment of squamous cervical intraepithelial neoplasia. *Int. J. Cancer,* 2006 Apr. 15; 118(8):2048-55.

[5]   Stokes-Lampard H., Wilson S., Waddell C., Ryan A., Holder R., Kehoe S. Vaginal vault smears after hysterectomy for reasons other than malignancy: a systematic review of the literature. *BJOG,* 2006 Dec.; 113(12):1354-65.

[6]   Stokes-Lampard H., Wilson S., Waddell C., Bentley L. Vaginal vault cytology tests: analysis of a decade of data from a UK tertiary centre. *Cytopathology,* 2011 Apr;22(2):121-9 doi: 10.1111/j.1365-2303.2010.00746.x. [Published online first 7 May 2010].

[7]   Strander B., Hällgren J., Sparén P. Effect of ageing on cervical or vaginal cancer in Swedish women previously treated for cervical intraepithelial neoplasia grade 3: population based cohort study of long

term incidence and mortality. *BMJ*, 2014 Jan. 14;348:f7361 doi: 10.1136/bmj.f7361.

[8] NHS Cervical Screening Programme. Colposcopy and Programme Management: Guidelines for the NHS Cervical Screening Programme 2010 http://www.cancerscreening.nhs.uk/cervical/publications/nhscsp20. html (accessed 26 June 2014).

[9] American College of Obstetricians and Gynaecologists. Screening for Cervical Cancer. Clinical management guideline No 131, 2012.

[10] Smith J. S., Backes D. M., Hoots B. E., Kurman R. J., Pimenta J. M. Human papillomavirus type-distribution in vulvar and vaginal cancers and their associated precursors. *Obstet. Gynecol.*, 2009 Apr.;113(4):917-24 doi: 10.1097/AOG.0b013e31819bd6e0.

[11] Zeligs K. P., Byrd K., Tarney C. M., Howard R. S., Sims B. D., Hamilton C. A., Stany M. P. A clinicopathologic study of vaginal intraepithelial neoplasia. *Obstet. Gynecol.*, 2013 Dec.;122(6):1223-30 doi: 10.1097/01.AOG.0000435450.08980.de.

[12] Katki H. A., Kinney W. K., Fetterman B., Lorey T., Poitras N. E., Cheung L., Demuth F., Schiffman M., Wacholder S., Castle P. E. Cervical cancer risk for women undergoing concurrent testing for humanpapillomavirus and cervicalcytology:a population based study in routine clinical practice. *Lancet Oncol.*, 2011 Jul.;12(7):663-72 doi: 10.1016/S1470-2045(11)70145-0. [Published online first 16 Jun 2011].

[13] Chao A., Chen T. C., Hsueh C., Huang C. C., Yang J. E., Hsueh S., Huang H. J., Lin C. T., Tang Y. H., Liou J. D., Chang C. J., Chou H. H., Lai C. H. Human papillomavirus in vaginal intraepithelial neoplasia. *Int. J. Cancer,* 2012 Aug. 1; 131(3):E259-68 doi: 10.1002/ijc.27354. [Published online first 14 Dec 2011].

In: Cryosurgery and Colposcopy
Editor: Lillian Watson

ISBN: 978-1-63484-507-6
© 2016 Nova Science Publishers, Inc.

Chapter 6

MANAGEMENT OF POSTCOITAL BLEEDING BETWEEN THE GENERAL GYNECOLOGY CLINIC AND COLPOSCOPY CLINIC

Fadi Alfhaily[1], and Ayman A. Ewies[2]*
[1]Consultant in Obstetrics and Gynaecology,
Colchester Hospital University NHS Foundation Trust, UK
[2]Consultant in Gynecology, Sandwell and West Birmingham Hospitals
NHS Trust, UK

ABSTRACT

Postcoital bleeding (PCB) is defined as spotting or bleeding that occurs during or after sexual intercourse unrelated to menstruation. It is a common gynecological symptom and is often alarming for women. The point prevalence of PCB determined in large community surveys ranges from 0.7 to 9% with an annual cumulative incidence of around 6% of menstruating women. Up to 5% of women are seen in a hospital's gynecology outpatient department due to PCB.

PCB could be the first sign of serious underlying pathology such as cervical intra-epithelial neoplasia (CIN), cervical carcinoma or chlamydial infection. It is estimated that the prevalence of cervical carcinoma and CIN in women with PCB varied between 0%-8% and

* Corresponding author: Fadi Alfhaily, MBChB, MSc, MRCOG, Consultant in Obstetrics and Gynaecology, Colchester Hospital University NHS Foundation Trust, UK Turner Road Colechester Essex CO45JL UK, Email: fadinm@yahoo.com & fadialfhaily@hotmail.com.

6.8%-19% respectively. It was reported that all symptomatic women with cervical carcinoma under 65 years of age had PCB. Moreover, PCB was found in 18%-38.3% of chlamydia- positive women.

There is great deal of controversy between gynecologists as regards managing women with PCB; probably due to the lack of well-designed studies and due to the variations in study design, including differences in symptom definition, time range in which the symptom occurred, frequency, age distribution of the population, and prevalence of sexually transmitted infection and use of hormones. Currently there are no well-defined guidelines available regarding how and where to manage these women. Many authors and experts recommend assessing women with PCB in the colposcopy clinic. However, other authors believe that, despite the well-reported association with serious pathology, referring every case of PCB for immediate investigation is inappropriate, impractical and not cost effective. This chapter will critically review the causes, risk factors and management of PCB in an attempt to outline a unified guidance based on the best available evidence for women and gynecologists alike.

BACKGROUND

Postcoital bleeding (PCB) is a common gynecological symptom that describes spotting or bleeding unrelated to menstruation that occurs during or after sexual intercourse. Although no underlying pathology is identified in 28.5-54.5% of cases [1, 2, 3], it could be a sign of serious pathology, such as cervical cancer, which is usually alarming and worrying for women. PCB most commonly develops in women aged 20 to 40 years and in those who are multiparous [3, 4].

28-39% of women with postcoital bleeding also experienced abnormal uterine bleeding, 13-15% had dyspareunia and 2.3% had vaginal discharge [5] [6, 3, 7].

The management of PCB varies and is inconsistent between gynecologists as there are no set of guidelines to ensure good practice.

EPIDEMIOLOGY AND PREVALENCE

While PCB is a common gynecological symptom, there is great disparity in determining the point prevalence in community populations. Earlier studies in 1960s and 1970s showed that in community population the calculated risk of cervical cancer in women with PCB was 1 in 220. [8] However, in a recent systematic review of 910 studies published in English the point prevalence of PCB ranged from 0.7% to 9% and 0.7 to 39% in general population and in women with cervical cancer, respectively [9]. Moreover, in a baseline cross sectional population survey followed by a prospective population-based cohort study of women using self-completed questionnaires about menstrual loss in a community population of a single general practice, PCB was reported in 6% (95% CI = 5 to 8) [10]. The same authors reported in a recent epidemiological study that the 2–year cumulative incidence of postcoital bleeding in naturally menstruating women was 7.7% (95% CI 6.2–9.5%). However, the rate of spontaneous resolution without recurrence for 2 years was 51% (95% CI 40–62). Of the 785 women identified with intermenstrual and/or postcoital bleeding, only one developed uterine cancer [11].

In secondary care, the point prevalence of PCB in new patients attending a hospital obstetrics and gynecology outpatients was reported to be 5% [12].

PATHOPHYSIOLOGY AND ETIOLOGY

Although the initial concern and fear for both patients and health care professionals is the possibility of underlying malignancy in women presenting with PCB, the majority of them will have benign causes.

PCB has multiple etiologies and the differential diagnosis is broad and wide. It is mainly caused by a surface lesion of the genital tract, such as cervical polyps, infection, ectropion, cervical intra epithelial neoplasia (CIN) or carcinoma [13].

The rate of no significant pathology in women with PCB varied between 15.1% and 67.2% [14] [15]. However, the rate of total significant pathology found in women with PCB was reported to vary between be 20.4% and 52.1% [1] [5].

Cancer

The great diversity in determining the prevalence of PCB in community populations raises concern about the usefulness of current guidelines, advising women when to consult based on symptoms, and the possibility of early detection of gynecological malignancy in the community and primary care. [10]. In his systematic review Shapely stated that the evidence base for the management strategies of postcoital bleeding and calculations of risk for cervical cancer in women with postcoital bleeding are poor. The calculation of risk for a woman seen in the community with postcoital bleeding and has cervical cancer ranges from 1 in 44 000 at age 20–24 years to 1 in 2400 aged 45–54 years. There was no information to allow the direct calculation of risk in women presenting to primary care [9].

Also, it was reported that all symptomatic women with cervical carcinoma under 65 years of age had PCB [16].

Moreover, the prevalence of cervical cancer and cervical intraepithelial neoplasia (CIN) in women presenting with PCB varied in different studies between 0% and 8% [1, 15, 17, 18, 19, 20] and 6.8% and 19% [3, 2, 15, 19, 21, 22] respectively. Whereas, PCB was reported as a presenting symptom in 6%–10% of women with cervical cancer [17, 18].

The PCB seen in these women is due to the fact that the epithelium associated with CIN and invasive cancer is thin, friable and readily detaches from the cervix.

The disparity in prevalence could be related to the different study designs and statistical analysis method used, different methodology, study geographical location, differences in symptom definition especially persistent PCB, time and frequency of PCB, age distribution of the population, prevalence of sexually transmitted infection and including women not having sexual relations in the study population.

Furthermore, endometrial cancer was reported in 0.3% of women presented with PCB [2, 14]; whereas vaginal cancer was reported in 0.3%-2.2% of cases [2, 21].

Table 1. shows the prevalence of cervical cancer and cervical intraepithelial neoplasia (CIN) in women presenting with PCB in different studies

Authors	Number	Design	Clinic setting	Pathology	
				Cancer	CIN
Shalini et al. (1998)	110	Retrospective analysis over 2 years	Colposcopy clinic	5.5%	Viral HPV and CIN I: 5.6% CIN II-III: 3.6%
2) Rosenthal et al. (2001)	314	Retrospective study over 6 years	General gynaecology service	4% in total: 3% cervical 0.6% endometrial 0.3% vaginal	Total: 17%: CIN II-III: 12% CIN I: 5% HPV: 6%

Authors	Number	Design	Clinic setting	Pathology	
				Cancer	CIN
Jha & Sabharwal (2002)	45	Retrospective Study over 1 year	Colposcopy	2.2%: invasive vaginal cancer	Total: 17.7% CIN I: 11.1% CIN II-III: 6.6%
Selo-Ojeme (2002)	248	Retrospectively reviewed the records of 248 patients over a 5-year	Gynecology and colposcopy clinics		CIN I: 10.1% CIN II-III:7.2% Overall incidence: 5%
Khattab et al. (2005)	284	Over eight years	Colposcopy and gynecology clinics	4.2% cervical, in both groups	32.7% had CIN in both groups
Abu et al. (2006)	142	A retrospective identification of cases from the computer over a period of 12 months	Colposcopy clinic	0	Total: 19% CIN II-III: 10.6%
Sahu et al. (2007)	87	Over 2 years	Negative cytology in the colposcopy unit	0	CIN I: 3.45% CIN II-III: 3.45%
Harry et al. (2007)	60	A prospective audit	Gynecology clinic or a colposcopy clinic	0	11% had CIN
Ray & Kaul (2008)	134 Only 64 had PCB	Retrospective study during the 24-month period	Colposcopy clinic with negative cytology		HPV: 24.3% LSIL: 5.4% HiSIL: 2.7% VAIN: 2.7%
Tehranian et al. (2009)	123	A cross-sectional study Over a 2-year period.		0.8% SCC 0.8% low grade CGIN	CIN I: 7.3% CIN II-III: 2.4%
Alfhaily & Ewies (2010)	137	A prospective observational non-comparative study between 1 September 2005 and 31 July 2009	Gynecology clinic or a colposcopy clinic	0.7%	13.1%
Obeidat and Saidi, (2012)	1470	A prospective study over 69 months	Colposcopy Clinic	0.4 cervical 0.3% endometrial	Total: 12.1% CIN II-III: 3.8% Low CGIN: 0.09% HPV: 14.4%
See AT & Havenga (2012)	73	1-year retrospective analysis	Colposcopy Clinic	1.4%	CIN: 15.1% HPV: 4.1%

Table 1. (Continued)

Authors	Number	Design	Clinic setting	Pathology	
				Cancer	CIN
Gulumser et al. (2015)	237	Retrospective cohort study. Between 2007 and 2013	Colposcopy Clinic		13.1%
Cheraghi et al. (2015)	50	A cross-sectional study between March 2013 and January 2014).	Colposcopy Clinic	2%	CIN I: 6% CIN II: 2%
Himanshi & lata (2015)	100	Prospective study from January 2007 to August 2008.	Gynae-Oncology unit followed by colposcopy clinic	8% invasive 2% in situ	LSIL: 6% HSIL: 9%

Infection

Many studies reported a link between persistent PCB and genital infection; PCB was found in 18–38% of women tested positive for Chlamydia [23, 24] and young women with PCB were found to be a high risk group for chlamydia therefore it was recommended that these women should be offered chlamydia screening [25].

The relative risk of chlamydial infection in women presenting with postcoital bleeding was found to be 2.6 times higher than that of a control group without bleeding [12].

In a prospective observational study chlamydia and bacterial vaginosis (BV) infection were found in 2.2% and 6.6% in women with PCB, respectively. The majority of women (81.8%) who had chlamydia and/or BV were over 35 years of age [1]. Also, Khattab et al. [26] found that 7.8% of women with PCB had chlamydia and 4.9% had BV.

However, despite the reported links between BV and postoperative infections especially vault haematomas after vaginal hysterectomy, endometritis, cervicitis and possibly pelvic inflammatory disease [27], the clinical significance of BV was not reported in majority of the studies. Moreover, BV was considered a risk factor for human immunodeficiency virus acquisition [28] and possibly CIN [29].

Chronic cervicitis was reported in 6.6% -36% in women presented with PCB [1, 4, 6, 20]; whereas acute cervicitis was found in 8% and ulcerative cervicitis in 4% [4, 6].

Table 2. The prevalence of infection in women presenting with PCB in different studies

Authors	Number	Pathology	
		STI/BV	**Other Infections**
Shalini et al. (1998)	110		21%
Khattab et al. (2005)	284	Chlamydia: 7.8% BV: 4.9%	
Sahu et al. (2007)	87	Chlamydia: 2.3% BV: 5.75%	
Ray & Kaul (2008)	64/134		Inflammation: 45.94%
Tehranian et al. (2009)	123		Chronic cervicitis: 31.7% Acute cervicitis: 8.1% Ulcerative cervicitis: 4.1%
Alfhaily & Ewies (2010)	137	Chlamydia: 2.2% BV: 6.6%	Cervicitis: 6.6%
See AT & Havenga (2012)	73		9.6% type
Cheraghi et al. (2015)	50		Chronic cervicitis: 36% Acute cervicitis: 8% Ulcerative cervicitis: 4%
Himanshi & lata (2015)	100		Chronic cervicitis: 29%

Cervical Ectropion

Cervical ectropion was the most common single finding in majority of the studies, it was reported in 25%-55% of cases [1, 15, 20, 26]; however 2 studies reported cervical ectropion only in 4.4% and 11.4% [6, 21].

Many authors do not considered cervical ectropion to be pathological in asymptomatic women; however, it is believed that we should not necessarily assume it is the cause of symptoms in women with PCB. Therefore, those with ectropion and PCB should be promptly referred for assessment [30].

The prevalence of ectropion increased with parity and decreased in women aged 35 and over when adjusted to other factors. Also, it was significantly more common in women taking oral contraceptives; however, it was less common in women using barrier methods [30].

Table 3. The rate of no pathology and other pathology in women presenting with PCB in different studies

Authors	Number	No pathology	Pathology		
			Ectropion	Other	Total pathology rate
Shalini et al. (1998)	110	67.2%			
Rosenthal et al. (2001)	314	49%		Cervical polyps: 5%	
Jha & Sabharwal (2002)	45		4.4%	Cervical polyps: 4.4%	20%
Selo-Ojeme (2002)	248		25.6%	Cervical polyps: 8.3% Endometrial polyps: 3.6% in total; 7.4% in hysteroscopy group Polyps and ectropion: 4.1%	
Khattab et al. (2005)	284	42.2- 85.6%	22.9-5.1%	Cervical polyps: 7.8-2.5% Cervical ulceration: 3.6-1.7%	
Abu et al. (2006)	142	39.4%	31%	Cervical polyps 4.9%	
Sahu et al. (2007)	87	52.4%	33.6%	Cervical polyps: 12.5%	
Harry et al. (2007)	60	38.3% Both groups	36.6% Both groups		
Ray & Kaul (2008)	134	28.1%	25%	Atrophic changes: 7.8% Cervical polyps: 10.9%	
Tahranian et al. (2007)	123		11.38%	Cervical polyps: 14.63%	
Alfhaily & Ewies (2010)	137	28.5%	45.3%	Atrophic changes: 5.8%	20.4%
Obeidat and Saidi, (2012)	1470	15.1%	25.2%		
See AT & Havenga (2012)	73	47.9%	19.2%	Cervical polyps: 2.7%	52.1%
Cheraghi et al. (2015)	50	22%		Cervical polyps: 16%	
Himanshi & lata (2015)	100		55%	Cervical polyps: 6%	

Other Pathology

Cervical polyps are not uncommon finding in women with PCB due to cervical trauma during intercourse. They are considered the most common benign neoplastic growth that occurs on the cervix with an incidence of 4% of gynecologic patients and typically occur in multiparous patients in their 40s to 50s. It is believed that they originate from recurrent inflammation of the cervix and/or cervix exposed to focal response to hormonal stimulation; and usually they are friable and bleed easily when touched [31].

They were reported in 2.2%-16% in women with PCB. [4, 5] and endometrial polyps were seen 1.45%-7.4% in women with PCB and IMB [1, 3].

Also, Atrophic changes were reported in 5.8%-7.8% cases [1, 32].

EVALUATION, STRATIFICATION OF RISK FACTORS AND DIAGNOSTIC WORKSHOP

The investigation for PCB bleeding depends on multiple risk factors, including duration of PCB, age, cervical smear history and smoking; based on these variables a gynecologist should be able to make a risk assessment of malignancy and formalise his plan of care.

In general, there is a lack of consensus about the pathways and algorithms of management of women with PCB; A questionnaire study included 1020 consultant gynecologists in the UK showed that there is a great deal of diversity in management of women with PCB amongst UK gynecologists; probably due to the lack of well-designed studies [33].

To date, there are no recommendations from the American College of Obstetricians and Gynecologists (ACOG), the Royal College of Obstetricians and Gynecologists (RCOG) or Society for Gynecologic Oncologists setting the standard of care for women with postcoital bleeding. Hence, the management is still inconsistent between gynecologists and there is uncertainty where and when to see these women.

Urgency of Referral

The Guidelines for Suspected Cancer published by the Department of Health (DoH), that set criteria for referral, recommended urgent referral (within 2 weeks) for women more than 35 years of age with PCB for more than 4 weeks, and early referral (within 4–6 weeks) in all other cases of repeated unexplained PCB [34]; the National Health Services Cervical Screening Programme (NHSCSP) increased the cut-off age to more than 40 years [35], whereas The Royal Australian College of Obstetricians and Gynaecologists and the Royal Australian College of General Practitioners (RANZCOG Statements) indicated that women complaining of postcoital bleeding (PCB) should have tests to exclude cervical cancer and Chlamydia [36].

Alfhaily & Ewies [1] found that only 6.5% women who had PCB for more than 4 weeks were referred urgently.

Age, Duration and Severity of PCB, Other Risk Factors

Many investigators disputed and questioned the validity of DoH guideline for referral as they found that the rate of pathology was not correlated to the women age [1, 3, 7, 26, 33] or the duration of PCB [15]. Nevertheless, 59.6% of the UK gynecologists agreed with it [33].

It was difficult to group the studies depending on the age of the women; this was due to the different ways that the authors have taken in measuring age. Only few studies provided data about the mean and range; other studies provided different age bands (Table 4).

In general, 50% of women who had significant pathology were less than 35 years of age and 92.8% had PCB for more than 4 weeks, whereas only 25% suffered severe episodes, suggesting that the duration of PCB, but not age or severity, is more important [1]. This was also supported by another prospective study of 100 women with postcoital bleeding and investigated by cytology, colposcopy and colposcopic directed biopsy of suspicious lesion; majority of the women had duration of postcoital bleeding 1-3 month; HiSIL and invasive cervical cancer were most common in women having post-coital bleeding more than 6 months duration (30% and 10% respectively); also 5 out 8 women how had invasive cancer were between 31-40 years old; with mean age 42.5 years [20] Similar findings were also reported by a retrospective analysis that showed the mean age for invasive cancer was 41.3 years and 32.9 years for benign pathologies [15].

Table 4. Distribution of age in women presenting PCB

Authors	N	Age						
		Mean	Median	Range	$\leq$30	31-40	41-50	>50
Rosenthal (2001)	314	34.4						
Selo-Ojeme (2002)	248			21-40	73	86	67	22
Khattab et al. (2005)	284				107	111	55	11
Cheraghi et al. (2015)	50	33.6			14	28	8	0
Abu et al. (2006)	102	34.1		16-61				
					<25	26-35	36-45	>45
Sahu et al. (2007)	87	37.5			6	31	32	18
					20-45	>45		
Tehranian (2009)	123	37.8			105	18		
					$\leq$35	36-40	>40	
Alfhaily & Ewies (2010)	137	38.17	38	18-65	48	19	51	
					<25	25-50	>50	
See AT & Havenga (2012)	73				17	52	4	
Himanshi & lata (2015)	100	34.5		22-62				

Furthermore, as the majority (81.8%) of women with PCB and positive chlamydia and/or BV were over 35 years of age [1], it might be inappropriate to exclude younger women with persistent PCB from rapid referral based on their age.

Not all studies recorded the same information regarding parity. Moreover, majority of them were retrospective, therefore, most authors were unable to analyze other demographic variables such as smoking, number of sexual partners and any previous history of sexually transmitted infections which could potentially influence the incidence of significant pathology in these women. Only one cohort retrospective study included 237 referred to the colposcopy clinic reported that only smoking, HPV and abnormal cytology increase the probability of CIN II or higher lesion by 1.686 times, 4.065 times and 5.787 times, respectively [37]. However, the regression analysis used in this study revealed only 33% of sensitively and 85% of specificity for the risk of CIN II or higher lesion; furthermore, authors were also unable to analyze all other risk factors such as number of sexual partners, previous history of sexually transmitted infections and amount of smoking.

Clinic setting

Currently, there arc many variations based on expert opinion about whether women with PCB should be referred for colposcopy or seen in general gynecological clinic; this uncertainty amongst gynecologists as to where women with PCB should be referred and seen could be influenced by multiple logistic factors within each unit e.g., access to colposcopy clinics, load of work and by the qualifications of the respondents e.g., being colposcopy trained. In the UK based survey inquiring about the current practice among 1020 consultants' gynecologists only 31.4% respondents believe that women ought to have colposcopy as a primary procedure, while only 16.7% actually see them in the colposcopy clinic [33].

If a woman has an abnormal smear or a grossly visible suspicious cervical lesion for underlying malignancy there is no doubt that she should be seen in colposcopy. However, there is debate and inconsistency about whether women with negative cervical smear and no visible lesions should be referred for colposcopy assessment.

Currently, PCB alone is not considered an absolute indication for referral to colposcopy in the most centres, and The National Health Services Cervical Screening Programme (NHSCSP) [35] recommended that women presenting with symptoms of cervical cancer – such as postcoital bleeding (particularly in women over 40 years), intermenstrual bleeding and persistent vaginal discharge – should be referred for gynecological examination and onward referral for colposcopy if cancer is suspected.

Examination should be performed by a gynecologist (such as a cancer lead gynecologist) experienced in the management of cervical disease. They should be seen urgently, within two weeks of referral. The programme recognises that although postcoital bleeding is a cardinal sign of cervical neoplasia, the majority of cases are not malignant, therefore in younger women, where chlamydial infection and problems with family planning are more likely causes, these women require appropriate assessment and referral for colposcopy if cancer is suspected [35].

In his systematic review Shapley stated that women need to be involved in decisions about their care and this involves communicating risk and an exploration of the implications of the risk. Moreover, women have the right to accept or refuse whatever is proposed and in taking a decision as to whether or not to investigate for underlying malignancy, informed consent is required [9].

A retrospective study of 314 women with postcoital bleeding seen by a gynecologic service found that 40% of women who had cancer had a normal smear before being referred for further investigation of postcoital bleeding, 20% of these cancers were visible only with the aid of the colposcopy. Therefore, 0.6% of women attending gynecology service with postcoital bleeding, a normal looking cervix and a normal smear had invasive cancer of the cervix [2]. Moreover, Sahu et al. [7] found that 6.9% of women had abnormal histology (two had CIN II) even though they had negative smears.

The Royal Australian College of Obstetricians and Gynaecologists and the Royal Australian College of General Practitioners stated clearly that it is commonly accepted that a single episode of PCB in a woman who has a normal smear and cervical appearance does not warrant immediate referral, but recurrence or persistence of this symptom mandates colposcopic examination [36]. This is supported by Jha and Sabharwal [21] in their 1-year audit as they found that if abnormal smears were the absolute referral criteria four women with cervical pathology would not have received colposcopy. Hence cytology would have missed 50% of the cases.

Therefore, many investigators and colposcopists [16, 20-22, 33, 38] believe that PCB should be an indication for referral to the colposcopy clinic; however, this is not the standard practice.

Cervical Smear

Many studies questioned the value of cytology alone in women with persistent PCB and reported that normal and inflammatory cytology alone did not guarantee a cervix free from dysplasia and concluded that colposcopy in combination with cytology permitted increased ability to detect CIN [38].

Table 5. Colposcopy, biopsy and smear findings in women with PCB

Authors	Design	Pathology linked to Smear, biopsy and colposcopy
Rosenthal et al. (2001)	Retrospective study over 6 years	• 30% of women with cervical cancer or CIN had a normal or inflammatory smear before being referred for further investigation of PCB
Jha & Sabharwal (2002)	Retrospective Study over 1 year	• 8.3% of women with PCB and negative referral smear had histological abnormalities confirmed by colposcopically directed biopsies
		• 24.2% of women with no referral smears were found to have histological abnormalities in colposcopically directed biopsies
		• If abnormal smears were the absolute referral criteria: four women with cervical pathology would not have received colposcopy; hence cytology alone would have missed 50% of the cases.
Khattab et al. (2005)	Over eight years	• the rate of cervical cancer and CIN was found to be 3.6% and 9%, respectively, in a review of the record of 166 women with PCB and normal smear history
Abu et al. (2006)	A retrospective identification of cases from the computer over a period of 12 months	• 19% of the 142 women referred to colposcopy primarily because of PCB, had CIN, mainly of high-grade, and most of them had a negative last cervical smear
Sahu et al. (2007)	Over 2 years	• 6.9% of women with PCB and normal smears had dysplasia on histology
Ray & Kaul (2008)	Retrospective study during the 24-month period	• 2.2% of women with negative smear had high-grade HiSIL which was determined after 66 biopsies.
Alfhaily & Ewies (2010)	A prospective observational non-comparative study	• the prevalence of CIN was 28.6% of those who were seen in colposcopy
		• 78.9% (15 out of 19) who had CIN and adenocarcinoma in situ had negative previous smear history

Alfhaily & Ewies reported in their prospective study of 137 women with PCB that the prevalence of CIN was 28.6% of those who were seen in colposcopy and 78.9% (15 out of 19) who had CIN and adenocarcinoma in situ had negative previous smear history. Also, Jha and Sabharwal [21] found that 8.3% of women with PCB and negative referral smear had histological abnormalities confirmed by colposcopically directed biopsies and 24.2% of women with no referral smears were found to have histological abnormalities in colposcopically directed biopsies. These finding were supported by many different studies [2, 7, 19, 26, 32].

In its statement the Royal Australian and New Zealand College of Obstetricians and Gynaecologists in 2004 stated that a normal smear should not be regarded as reassuring in women with persistent PCB and recommended repeating the smear if it was taken more than 3 months before the episode. However, Woodman et al. [39] found that majority of GPs (89%) and majority of family planning doctors (86%) will repeat the smear in women with PCB and normal smear only if it was done 18 months before referral.

Moreover, in their survey, Alfhaily & Ewies [33] reported that only 48.8% respondents repeat the cervical smear for only those with negative smear history who are still within the national screening interval; 36.7% repeat it only if it was done >12 months before the episode of PCB, 36.4% repeat it if it was done >6 months, and 21.8% repeat it if it was done >3 months.

Table 5 shows the colposcopy, biopsy and smear findings in women with PCB between these studies.

Genital Swabs

Despite the well-reported link between infection and persistent PCB [1, 23, 24, 26] only 58.9%, 65.8% and 79.8% of UK consultant will consider doing high vaginal swabs, endocervical swabs and chlamydia swabs, respectively to investigate for women with persistent PCB [33]. This may reflect underestimating and undermining the significance of the problem. Many investigators [23, 25, 40, 41] found that the PCB was reported in 21.3%, 33.3%, 10.5% and 9.4% respectively in women tested positive for chlamydia (Table 6).

Cervical infection was reported as a significant finding in many studies [1, 4, 6, 20]; therefore it is important to screen women with PCB and treat any infection as early as possible to prevent significant complications such as pelvic inflammatory disease, increased risk of ectopic pregnancy, subfertility and chronic pelvic pain.

Cervicitis is an inflammation of the cervical stroma and can be acute or chronic. Infected women were more likely to be younger, to have spotting or postcoital bleeding, to have a mucoid or purulent cervical discharge and to have signs of cervical inflammation, especially friability [23]. Acute cervicitis may be caused by infection with *C. trachomatis, N. gonorrhea, T. vaginalis, G. vaginalis*, and mycoplasma species. Chronic cervicitis usually does not have an infectious source [23].

Table 6. The prevalence of PCB in women tested positive for chlamydia

	Linder et al., 1998	Verhoeven et al., 2003	Gotz et al., 2005	Chen et al., 2005
Design	Prospective	Prospective	Prospective	Retrospective
No. tested	439	787	4304	340
No. +ve for chalmydia	61	5%	114	170
No. -ve for chalmydia	432		4190	170
PCB in Chlamydia +ve	13	33.3%	12	16
PCB in Chlamydia -ve	33		184	6

Other Investigations

Majority of the gynecologists do not consider investigating the endometrium despite the reported link between PCB and endometrial pathology such as endometrial polyps, endometritis or cancer. Although this is less common, it could be relevant in women with persistent PCB or those with mixed PCB and IMB [2, 3, 13]. Only 27.3%, 16.5% and 12.1% of UK consultant gynecologists consider pelvic ultrasound scan, pipelle endometrial sample and hysteroscopy, respectively in cases of persistent PCB and/or in those with associated intermenstrual bleeding (IMB) [33].

Nonetheless, more trials and research are needed to explore this area further and determine whether there is a certain age limit above which the endometrium should be investigated [33].

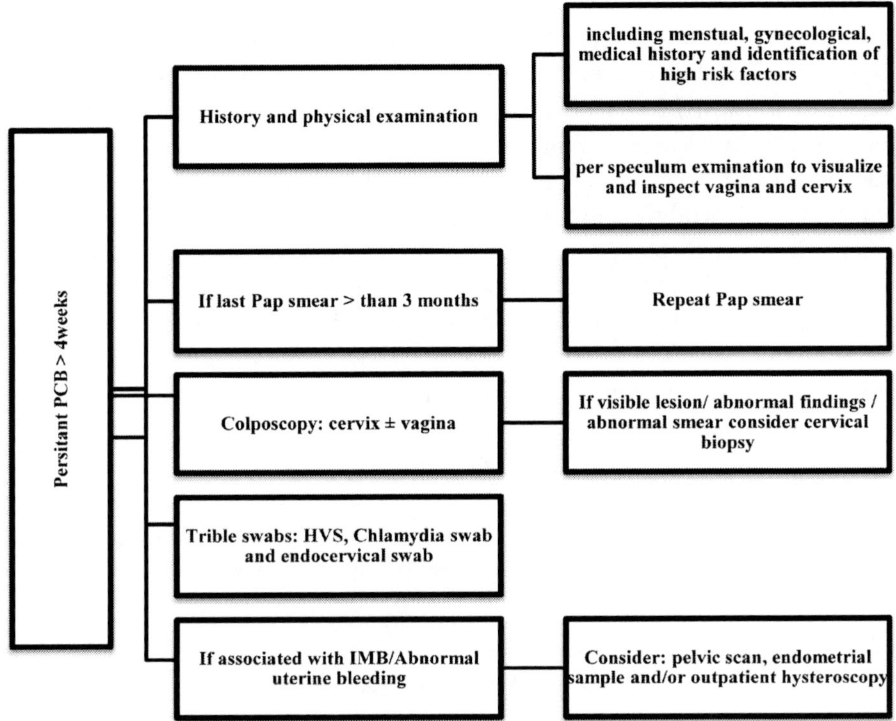

Figure 1. Evaluation and diagnostic workshop of PCB.

SUMMARY AND RECOMMENDATION

To date, and unlike heavy menstrual bleeding, abnormal uterine bleeding, postmenopausal bleeding or the management of abnormal cytology, there are no guidelines or clear recommendation from any organisation or governing body on the management of women presenting persistent postcoital bleeding. A full gynecological history and physical/pelvic examination is required to guide evaluation and develop a differential diagnosis. Although majority of women presenting with postcoital bleeding will not have underlying malignancy, significant pathology is much commoner in these women than the general population, therefore primary and secondary health care providers should take the appropriate screening tests. We recommend that women with PCB for more than 4 weeks should have: full and comprehensive history taking including stratification of risk factors, pelvic examination, smear testing (if the previous one was done more than 3 months before consultation), triple swabs (chlamydial, endocervical and high vaginal) and colposcopy. If PCB is associated with IMB/PMB other investigation such as pelvic scan, endometrial biopsy and/or hysteroscopy should be considered. (Figure 1) Clinicians should build up an effective risk communication and shared decision making with their patients depending on multiple different risk factors that may vary from doctor-oriented expectation to patient centred expectation; strategies, clear protocols and pathways should be readily available to promote the concept of shared decision making and then clear and easy referral. Also, clinicians should have all the needed support to make clear estimation of the positive predictive factors and values of postcoital bleeding in relation to cervical cancer and/or other significant pathology to enable formalising clear pathways in decision making in primary care when investigating women with symptoms that might suggest risk of cervical cancer.

Research and further large multi-centre studies are required to provide more information that could help in optimising the management of PCB.

REFERENCES

[1]   Alfhaily, F; Ewies, AA. Managing women with post-coital bleeding: a prospective observational non-comparative study. *J Obstet Gynaecol.*, 2010 Feb, 30(2), 190-4.

[2]   Rosenthal, AN; Panoskaltsis, T; Smith, T; Soutter, WP. The frequency of significant pathology in women attending a general gynaecological service for postcoital bleeding. *Bjog.*, 2001 Jan, 108(1), 103-6.

[3]   Selo-Ojeme, DO; Dayoub, N; Patel, A; Metha, M. A clinico-pathological study of postcoital bleeding. *Archives of gynecology and obstetrics.*, 2004 Jul, 270(1), 34-6.

[4]   Fateme Cheraghi, PJ; Kambiz, Masoumi; Arash, Forouzan; Razieh, Mohamad Jafari. Comparison Results of Pap Smear and Colposcopy and Histopathology in Women with Post-Coital Bleeding. *Research Journal of Obstetrics and Gynecology.*, 2015, 8(1), 10-5.

[5]   See, AT; Havenga, S. Outcomes of women with postcoital bleeding. *International journal of gynaecology and obstetrics: the official organ of the International Federation of Gynaecology and Obstetrics.*, 2012 Jan, 120(1), 88-9.

[6]   Tehranian, A; Rezaii, N; Mohit, M; Eslami, B; Arab, M; Asgari, Z. Evaluation of women presenting with postcoital bleeding by cytology and colposcopy. *International journal of gynaecology and obstetrics: the official organ of the International Federation of Gynaecology and Obstetrics.*, 2009 Apr, 105(1), 18-20.

[7]   Sahu, B; Latheef, R; Aboel Magd, S. Prevalence of pathology in women attending colposcopy for postcoital bleeding with negative cytology. *Archives of gynecology and obstetrics.*, 2007 Nov, 276(5), 471-3.

[8]   Hakama, M; Joutsenlahti, U; Virtanen, A; Rasanen-Virtanen, U. Mass screenings for cervical cancer in Finland 1963-71. Organization, extent, and epidemiological implications. *Annals of clinical research.*, 1975 Apr, 7(2), 101-11.

[9]   Shapley, M; Jordan, J; Croft, PR. A systematic review of postcoital bleeding and risk of cervical cancer. *Br J Gen Pract.*, 2006 Jun, 56(527), 453-60.

[10]   Shapley, M; Jordan, K; Croft, PR. An epidemiological survey of symptoms of menstrual loss in the community. *Br J Gen Pract.*, 2004 May, 54(502), 359-63.

[11]   Shapley, M; Blagojevic-Bucknall, M; Jordan, KP; Croft, PR. The epidemiology of self-reported intermenstrual and postcoital bleeding in the perimenopausal years. *Bjog.*, 2013 Oct, 120(11), 1348-55.

[12]   Bax, CJ; Oostvogel, PM; Mutsaers, JA; Brand, R; Craandijk, M; Trimbos, JB; et al. Clinical characteristics of Chlamydia trachomatis infections in a general outpatient department of obstetrics and gynaecology in the Netherlands. *Sexually transmitted infections.*, 2002 Dec, 78(6), E6.

[13]   Fraser, IS; Petrucco, OM. Management of intermenstrual and postcoital bleeding, and an appreciation of the issues arising out of the recent case of O'Shea versus Sullivan and Macquarie pathology. *The Australian & New Zealand journal of obstetrics & gynaecology.*, 1996 Feb, 36(1), 67-73.

[14]   Saidi, RAOaSA. Prevalence of High-Grade Cervical Intraepithelial Neoplasia (CIN) and Cervical Cancer in Women with Post-Coital Bleeding (PCB) and Negative Smear: A Retrospective Study. *Gynecologic and obstetric investigation.*, 2012, 2.

[15]   Shalini, R; Amita, S; Neera, MA. How alarming is post-coital bleeding-- a cytologic, colposcopic and histopathologic evaluation. *Gynecologic and obstetric investigation.*, 1998, 45(3), 205-8.

[16] Slater, DN. Multifactorial audit of invasive cervical cancer: key lessons for the National Screening Programme. *Journal of clinical pathology.*, 1995 May, 48(5), 405-7.

[17] Pardanani, NS; Tischler, LP; Brown, WH; Feo, ED. Carcinoma of cervix. Evaluation of treatment in community hospital. *New York state journal of medicine.*, 1975 Jun, 75(7), 1018-21.

[18] Pretorius, R; Semrad, N; Watring, W; Fotheringham, N. Presentation of cervical cancer. *Gynecologic oncology.*, 1991 Jul, 42(1), 48-53.

[19] Abu, J; Davies, Q; Ireland, D. Should women with postcoital bleeding be referred for colposcopy? *J Obstet Gynaecol.*, 2006 Jan, 26(1), 45-7.

[20] Dr. Gangwal Himanshi, DRL. Evaluation of Post Coital Bleeding By Cinical and Pathalogical Finding. *IOSR Journal of Dental and Medical Sciences (IOSR-JDMS).* Aug. 2015, 14(8 Ver. III), 31-4.

[21] Jha, S; Sabharwal, S. Outcome of colposcopy in women presenting with postcoital bleeding and negative or no cytology--results of a 1-year audit. *J Obstet Gynaecol.*, 2002 May, 22(3), 299-301.

[22] Anorlu, RI; Abdul-Kareem, FB; Abudu, OO; Oyekan, TO. Cervical cytology in an urban population in Lagos, Nigeria. *J Obstet Gynaecol.*, 2003 May, 23(3), 285-8.

[23] Lindner, LE; Geerling, S; Nettum, JA; Miller, SL; Altman, KH. Clinical characteristics of women with chlamydial cervicitis. *The Journal of reproductive medicine.*, 1988 Aug, 33(8), 684-90.

[24] Nher, H; Lamminger, C; Zimmermann, J; Petzoldt, D. [The value of symptoms and clinical findings in cervical Chlamydia trachomatis infection]. *Der Hautarzt; Zeitschrift fur Dermatologie, Venerologie, und verwandte Gebiete.*, 1991 Nov, 42(11), 687-91.

[25] Gotz, HM; van Bergen, JE; Veldhuijzen, IK; Broer, J; Hoebe, CJ; Steyerberg, EW; et al. A prediction rule for selective screening of Chlamydia trachomatis infection. *Sexually transmitted infections.*, 2005 Feb, 81(1), 24-30.

[26] Khattab, AF; Ewies, AA; Appleby, D; Cruickshank, DJ. The outcome of referral with postcoital bleeding (PCB). *J Obstet Gynaecol.*, 2005 Apr, 25(3), 279-82.

[27] Sweet, RL. Gynecologic conditions and bacterial vaginosis: implications for the non-pregnant patient. *Infectious diseases in obstetrics and gynecology.*, 2000, 8(3-4), 184-90.

[28] Myer, L; Kuhn, L; Stein, ZA; Wright, TC; Jr. Denny, L. Intravaginal practices, bacterial vaginosis, and women's susceptibility to HIV

infection: epidemiological evidence and biological mechanisms. *The Lancet.*, 2005 Dec, 5(12), 786-94.

[29] Platz-Christensen, JJ; Sundstrom, E; Larsson, PG. Bacterial vaginosis and cervical intraepithelial neoplasia. *Acta obstetricia et gynecologica Scandinavica.*, 1994 Aug, 73(7), 586-8.

[30] Goldacre, MJ; Loudon, N; Watt, B; Grant, G; Loudon, JD; McPherson, K; et al. Epidemiology and clinical significance of cervical erosion in women attending a family planning clinic. *British medical journal.*, 1978, Mar 25, 1(6115), 748-50.

[31] Farrar, HK; Jr. Nedoss, BR. Benign tumors of the uterine cervix. *American journal of obstetrics and gynecology.*, 1961 Jan, 81, 124-37.

[32] Ray, P; Kaul, V. Prevalence of high-grade squamous intraepithelial neoplasia (HiSIL) in symptomatic women referred to the colposcopy clinic with negative cytology. *Archives of gynecology and obstetrics.*, 2008 Jun, 277(6), 501-4.

[33] Alfhaily, F; Ewies, AA. Postcoital bleeding: a study of the current practice amongst consultants in the United Kingdom. *European journal of obstetrics, gynecology, and reproductive biology.*, 2009 May, 144(1), 72-5.

[34] Department of Health, D. Department of Health. *Referral guidelines for suspected cancer*, 2000, p. 25. 2000.

[35] NHS Cervical Screening Programme Second edition N. Colposcopy and programme management Guidelines for the NHS Cervical Screening Programme Second edition NHSCSP Publication No 20 May 2010. 2010.

[36] RANZCOG Statements. Investigation of intermenstrual and postcoital bleeding. http://wwwranzcogeduau/component/docman/doc_details/907-investigation. 2012.

[37] Gulumser, C; Tuncer, A; Kuscu, E; Ayhan, A. Is colposcopic evaluation necessary in all women with postcoital bleeding? *European journal of obstetrics, gynecology, and reproductive biology.*, 2015 Oct, 193, 83-7.

[38] Harahap, RE. Combination of cytology and colposcopy in diagnosis of cervical intraepithelial neoplasia. *Cancer detection and prevention.*, 1981, 4(1-4), 461-4.

[39] Woodman, CB; Richardson, J; Spence, M. Why do we continue to take unnecessary smears? *Br J Gen Pract.*, 1997 Oct, 47(423), 645-6.

[40] Verhoeven, V; Avonts, D; Meheus, A; Goossens, H; Ieven, M; Chapelle, S; et al. Chlamydial infection: an accurate model for opportunistic screening in general practice. *Sexually transmitted infections.*, 2003 Aug, 79(4), 313-7.

[41] Chen, MY; Rohrsheim, R; Donovan, B. Chlamydia trachomatis infection in Sydney women. *The Australian & New Zealand journal of obstetrics & gynaecology.*, 2005 Oct, 45(5), 410-3.

Chapter 7

PHOTODYNAMIC THERAPY UNDER COLPOSCOPY FOR CIN AND EARLY STAGE UTERINE CERVICAL CANCER PRESERVING FERTILITY

Masaru Sakamoto[1,2], Noriko Yamaguchi[1,2], Keiji Morimoto[1,2], Kiyohiko Miyake[1], Yasuko Koyamatsu[1], Tetsuya Muroya[3], Tadao Tanaka[1] and Aikou Okamoto[2]

[1]Sasaki Foundation Kyoundo Hospital, Dept. of Gynecology, Tokyo, Japan
[2]Jikei University School of Medicine, Dept. of OB/GY, Tokyo, Japan
[3]Kokoro to Karada no Genki Plaza, Dept. of Gynecology, Tokyo, Japan

ABSTRACT

The number of the patient with dysplasia and CIS of the uterine cervix has been increasing recently, especially in the younger ages who need fertility preservation. Although cervical conization is standard therapy for dysplasia and CIS, the significant increase in the obstetrical risks such as premature delivery after conization has been reported. On the other hand, PDT is an excellent procedure to treat dysplasia and CIS by photochemical reaction generated by laser irradiation to the lesion under colposcopy after injection of tumor-specific photosensitizer. We have developed protocol and colposcope specifically designed to PDT, and applied PDT to dysplasia and CIS for 20 years. PDT was performed for 520 cases (146 dysplasia, 342 CIS, 4 AIS, 24 MIC, 1 MIAC, 2 invasive SCC, and 1 invasive adenoca.). 97% (503/520) of PDT cases were CR by the first PDT. 8 out of 16 PR cases turned out to be CR by the second PDT. CR rates for dysplasia, CIS, MIC were 99%, 97%, and 92%, respectively. These data suggest that PDT using colposcopy enables accurate LASER irradiation to uterine cervix resulting in high cure rate for CIN and early stage cervical cancer, and PDT for CIN and early stage uterine cervical cancer could be one of modalities of uterine preservation therapy as well as endocervical conization.

INTRODUCTION

Standard therapy for CIN (Cervical Intra-epithelial Neoplasia) and MIC (Micro invasive Ca.) is endo-cervical conization [1].

However, endocervical conization increases obstetrical risks such as PROM, premature delivery and low birth-weight due to the shortened cervical length [2].

On the other hand, PDT treats cancer using photodynamic reaction induced by tumor-specific photosensitizer when exposed to laser. Mechanism of PDT includes reactive oxygen generated by photochemical reaction, vascular shut down effect and induction of apoptosis [3, 4]. Free radicals such as reactive oxygen generated by photochemical reaction result in degeneration by oxidizing miniature organs within the malignant cells to manifest its ability to kill cells. Vascular shut-down effect due to the obstruction of endothelial cells within the neo blood vessels of tumor cells.

We have developed Photofrin PDT protocol for CIN and MIC using Excimer dye laser [5]. We have performed PDT for more than 500 cases of CIN and early stage cervical cancer with CR rate of 97%. Yamaguchi S, et al. reported PDT for 105 cases of CIN with CR rate of 90% [6].

PDT guideline for cervical lesion in Japan was published [7].

OBJECTIVES

At first, we report here clinical procedure, therapeutic effect, and prognosis after PDT for the CIN and early stage cervical cancer.

Secondly, we discuss about the advantages and disadvantages of PDT in comparison with laser vaporization and endocervical conization for CIN and early stage cervical cancer.

MATERIALS AND METHODS

Photosensitizer: Photofrin

Tumor affinity photosensitive substance: Porphyrin dimer to octomer mixed substance. Main component is dimer DHE (dehematoporphyrin ester/ether) a drug of freeze-dried powder consistency with a dark red color containing 75 mg Photofrin per vial (provided by Pfizer (Japan), Ltd.).

Laser Delivery Systems: Excimer Dye Laser (EDL) and YAG-OPO Laser

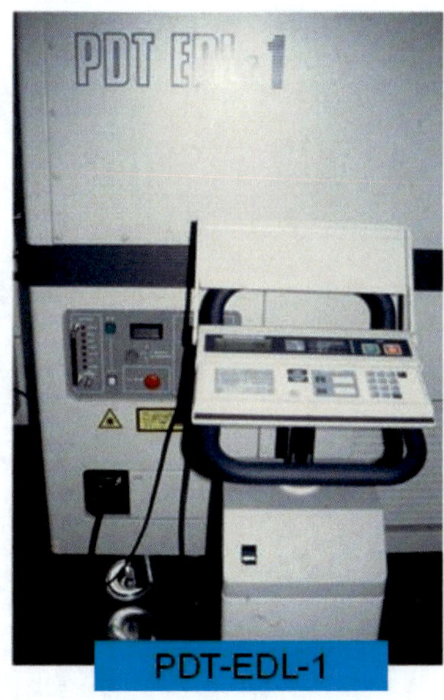

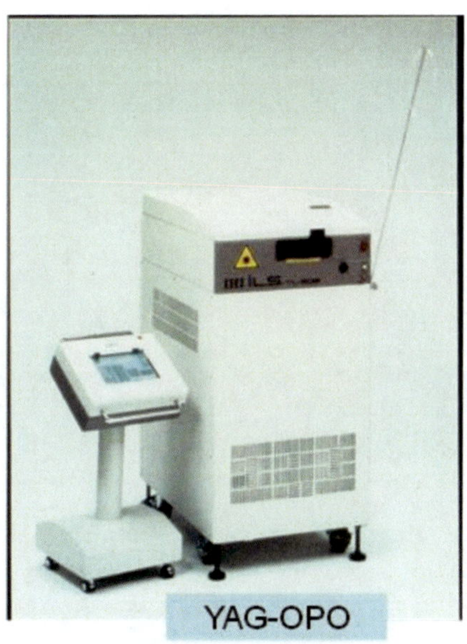

Figure 1. This figure shows two types of laser systems used for PDT. The left one is called as Excimer Dye Laser produced by Hamamatsu Photonics. The right one is called YAG-Optic Parametric Oscilator Laser produced by IHI. We have been mainly using Excimer Dye Laser.

The EDL is a low energy power laser, and its 630 nm wavelength dye laser is generated when rhodamine 640 pigment solution is irradiated by 308 nm ultra-violet rays generated by an XeCl Excimer laser. The laser wavelength is 630−635 nm, width of pulse is 10±5 nsec, and pulse radiation energy is 4−5 mJ/pulse maximum. Pulse repeated frequency is 40 Hz in normal cases (Figure 1 Left).

YAG-OP0 laser is a PDT laser that has an optic parametric oscillator (OPO), Q switch pulse YAG laser intensifier installed. Laser wave is 620 - 670nm, pulse width is 7 ± 1 nsec, pulse irradiation energy is 6 mJ/pulse, and repeated frequency is 50 Hz (Figure 1 Right).

Colposcope for Laser Therapy

A feature of the 0lympus Laser Colposcope is an optical path for the laser and allows cervical lesions to be examined during photoirradiation. With this method it is possible to show a 10 mm circular spot at the focus where the observation is made. This results in stable and precise photoirradiation (Figure 2).

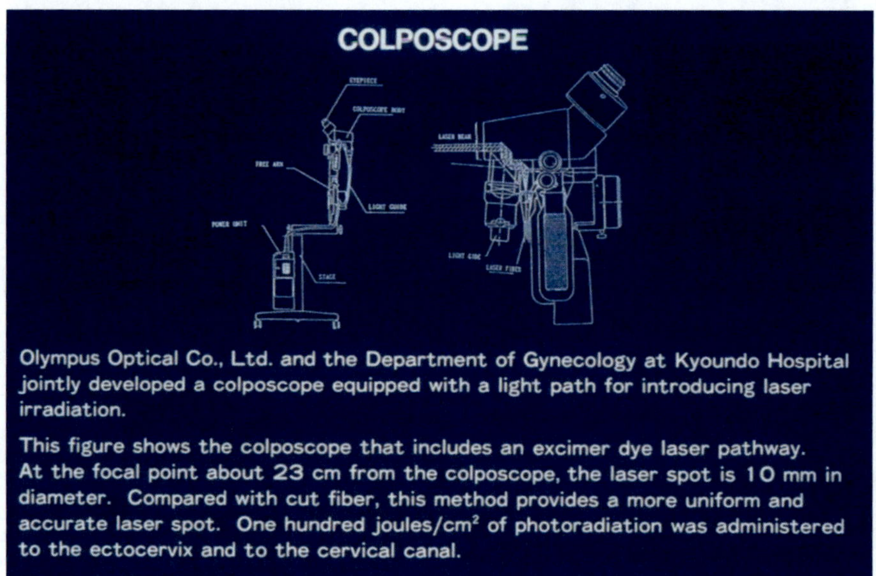

Olympus Optical Co., Ltd. and the Department of Gynecology at Kyoundo Hospital jointly developed a colposcope equipped with a light path for introducing laser irradiation.

This figure shows the colposcope that includes an excimer dye laser pathway. At the focal point about 23 cm from the colposcope, the laser spot is 10 mm in diameter. Compared with cut fiber, this method provides a more uniform and accurate laser spot. One hundred joules/cm^2 of photoradiation was administered to the ectocervix and to the cervical canal.

Figure 2.

Cervical Probe

This probe was developed to administer PDT in the cervical canal, i.e., endocervix. A special sapphire chip or ceramic chip is mounted on the tip of the cut fiber (Figure 3).

Cervical Probe Manipulator

Previously, the operator needed to mark the position where the cervical probe was originally inserted in order to withdraw in 1 mm increments. Presently, a cervical probe manipulator is installed in the colposcope, and it can move 0.5 mm in half revolutions and 1 mm in one complete revolution. This enables the operator to withdraw exactly 1 mm (Figure 3).

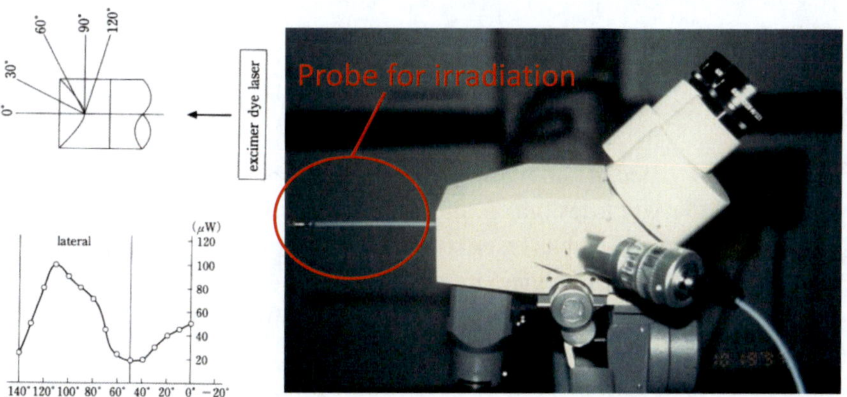

Figure 3. The Olympus Laser Colposcope features two optical paths for the laser. One is for colposcopic photoradiation by which 10 mm circular spot can be irradiated at the focus. Another optical path is for cervical probe which can treat cervical canal lesion efficiently. A concaved saphire chip is mounted on the tip of the cut fiber. The left figure shows the Laser power distribution of the cervical probe., indicating that 70% of the laser light is scattered to the side wall of the cervical canal.

Laser Power Distribution of the Cervical Probe

It can administer photoirradiation in a forward direction on the cervical canal side walls: 70% of the laser light is scattered to the side walls and 30% of the laser light forward. Thus, all of the cervical canal can be irradiated (Figure 4).

Classification by Colposcopic Findings

According to the location of the lesions on the uterine cervix, the results of PDT are divided into the following three types:

- Type I means that the second S−C Junction was visible.
- Type II means that the second S−C Junction was not visible.
- Type III means Uncertifiable Colposcopic Findings.

As a rule, Type III cases were excluded from PDT because the irradiation would have been blind.

Colposcope Irradiation (Spot Irradiation) (Figure 4)

1. Lesions located at the uterine cervix should be irradiated, particularly around the worst lesions at an energy intensity rate of 100 J/cm2 per shot using an Olympus laser colposcope through direct observation.
2. A large amount of cervical mucus is produced by irradiation. It should be removed using swabs or a 1 cc syringe for cervical mucus extraction whenever needed.
3. Spot irradiation should overlap without leaving retention on the circumference. The pattern should resemble Olympic Game logo.
4. Typically parts, uneven surfaces and angles such as the cervical canal, should be irradiated in all directions by carefully adjusting the Cusco speculum and changing the laser angle. (Especially when glandular involvement exists, irradiation needs to be thorough as it tends to leave areas which have not been irradiated in such case).

Materials and Methods

Patients: 520 cases of CIN and early stage cervical cancer

     ① 488 CIN (146 dysplasia + 342 CIS)

     ② 4 AIS   ② 25 cases of stage Ia cervical cancer

     ④ 3 cases of stage Ib1 cervical cancer

Photosensitizer: Photofrin 2mg/kg i.v.

Excimer-dye LASER irradiation:

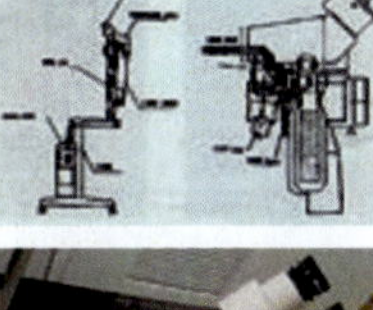
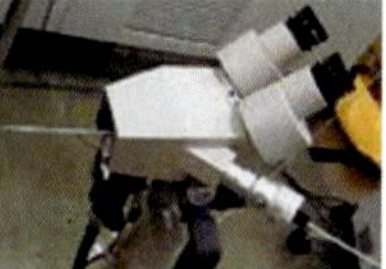

   ① colposcopic irradiation

   ② endocervical irradiation with a cervical probe

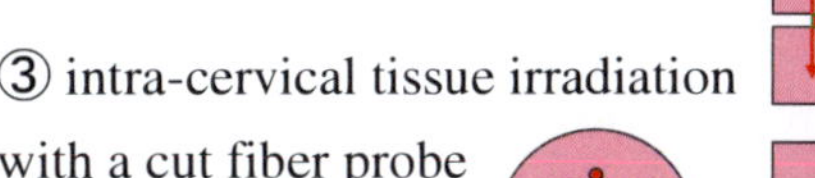
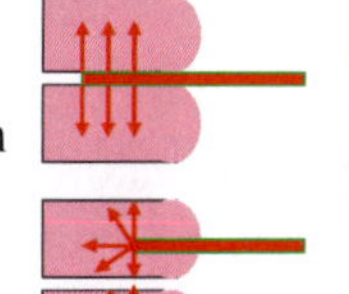

   ③ intra-cervical tissue irradiation

   with a cut fiber probe

Figure 4. PDT was performed with informed consent to 520 cases of CIN and early stage cervical cancer. The excimer-dye laser irradiation was performed using colposcopy and endocervical probe at 100J/cm2 48 hours after intra-venous administration of Photofrin at 2mg/kg. In addition to colposcopic and endocervical irradiation, for one case of residual cervical cancer with positive surgical margin after conization for microinvasive adenocarcinoma +CIS, intra-cervical tissue irradiation was performed by inserting a cut fiber into the portion from four separate sites around uterine external opening.

Cervical Canal Irradiation (Figure 4)

After confirming the lesion is inside the cervical canal by using a hysteroscope, the cervical probe should be inserted to the required depth. Irradiation should be repeated as the inserted fiber is drawn from the cervical canal in 1 mm increments till it drops out from the external uterine orifice.

Administration of Patients after Photofrin Injection

Patients become extremely sensitive to sunshine for about a week after Photofrin injection. When exposed to intense light, the exposed skin reddens and may develop optic hyperesthesia such as edema. Therefore, the patient's room brightness should be measured using a lux meter and the following adjustments should be observed:

Evaluation of Effectiveness of PDT

Two-three months after PDT patients are checked by cytological, colposcopic, histopathological findings, and they are divided into the following four levels.

Patients classified below PR are re-examined four-six months after PDT:

- CR: All lesions are completely cured in terms or cytological, colposcopic, and histopathological findings.
- PR: Almost all lesions are cured, but cytological, colposcopic, and histopathological findings suggest that some lesions may not yet be cured.
- NC: Most lesions are not cured, and cytological, colposcopic, and histopathological findings before PDT and after PDT are almost the same. Lesions from pre-PDT are completely preserved.
- PD: Among cytological, colposcopic,and histopathological findings, more than one finding became worse than before PDT.

RESULTS

There are colposcopic findings of three clinical samples treated by PDT.

Colposcopic findings before and after PDT for the first case of CIS was shown in Figure 5. Upper slides show colposcopic findings of CIS before PDT on the left indicating W1G0, and three months after PDT on the right side. Lower slides show colposcopic findings of CIS one year after PDT on the left, and two years after PDT on the right side, indicating the presense of normal gland openings.

Colposcopic findings before and after PDT for the second case of CIS and MIC were shown in Figure 6. Upper slides show colposcopic findings of CIS before PDT on the left indicating W1, and six weeks after PDT on the right side. Lower slides show colposcopic findings of MIC before PDT on the left indicating W2, and six months after PDT on the right side. Both cases showed that all abnormal colposcopic findings have completely disappeared after PDT.

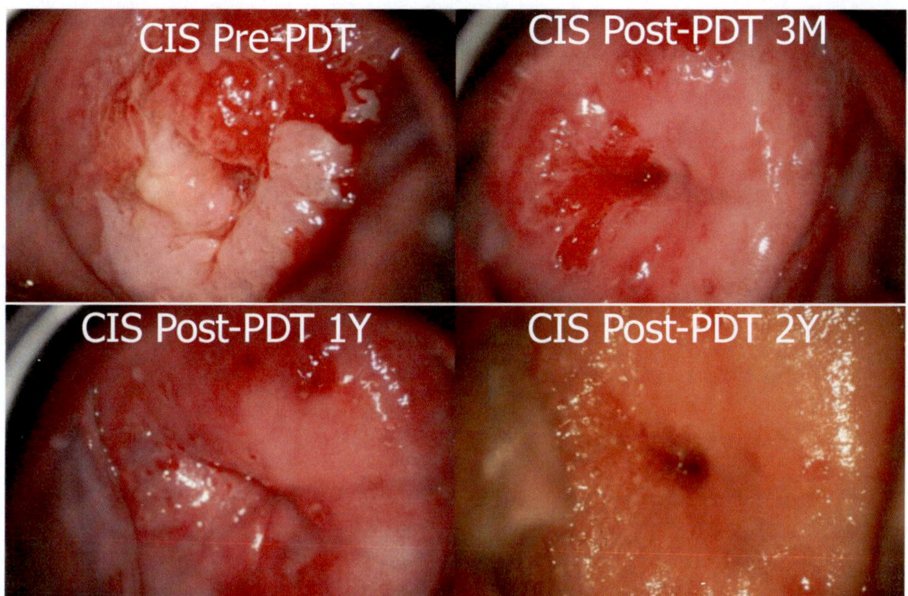

Figure 5.

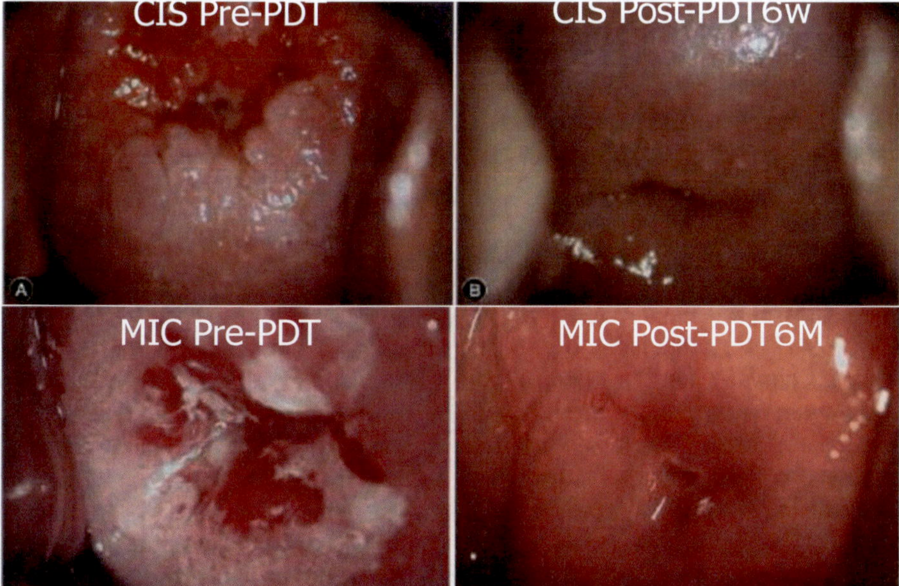

Figure 6.

We have developed protocol and colposcope specifically designed to PDT, and applied PDT to dysplasia and CIS for more than 20 years. Table 1 is a summary showing clinical response of PDT at Kyoundo Hospital since 1989 through 2007.

PDT was performed for 520 cases (146 dysplasia, 342 CIS, 4 AIS, 24 MIC, 1 MIAC, 2 invasive SCC, and 1 invasive adenoca).

97% (503/520) of PDT cases were CR by the first PDT. 8 out of 16 PR cases turned out to be CR by the second PDT. CR rates for dysplasia, CIS, MIC were 99%, 97%, and 92%, respectively.

Totally, 520 cases of cervical lesions have been treated by PDT. CR rate was 97 percent.

Table 1. Clinical response of PDT at Kyoundo Hospital (1989~2007)

	Case	CR	(%)	PR	(%)	NC	(%)
Dysplasia	146	144	98.6	2	1.4	0	0
CIS	342	330	96.5	11	3.2	1	0.3
		+ 8*		- 8*			
		338	98.8	3	0.9		
AIS	4	4	100	0	0	0	0
SCC Ia	24	22	91.7	2	8.3	0	0
SCC Ib	2	1	50	1	50	0	0
EC-Ad-Ca Ia	1	1	100	0	0	0	0
EC-Ad-Ca Ib	1	1	100	0	0	0	0
VAIN	5	5	100	0	0	0	0
VIN	3	3	100	0	0	0	0
Total	**528**	**511**	**96.8**	**16**	**3.0**	**1**	**0.2**
		+8*		-8*			
		519	98.3	8	1.5		

* 8 PR cases became CR after 2nd PDT.
VAIN: Vaginal Intraepithelial Neoplasia, VIN: Vulvar Intraepithelial Neoplasia.

Additional Therapy for 16 PR Cases

There were 16 PR cases after PDT. Additional therapy for 16 PR cases was performed as follows. In the case of residual Sever Dysplasia after PDT for CIN3, 3 out of 16 PR cases (18.8%) were under observation. Spontaneous regression was observed in 2 out of 3 cases. In the case of residual CIS after PDT for CIN3, 8 out of 16 PR cases (50%) underwent second PDT, resulting in CR in all 8 cases. Three out of 16 PR cases (18.8%) underwent endocervical conization, resulting in two cases with CR and one case with invasive cancer (Ib"occ"), followed by radical hysterectomy. One out of 16 PR cases (6.3%) who did not hope conization or PDT underwent RALS. In the PR case for cervical cancer stage Ib1, MIC was residual and trachelectomy after conization was performed.

Therapy for 7 Cases of Recurrence after CR (Table 2)

Seven out of 511 cases followed up for 16 through 234 months after PDT were found to be recurrent. Recurrent rate was 7 out of 511 cases, 1.4%. Recurrence as SD after PDT for SD was observed in 2 out of 7 cases (29%) 8 and 28 months later. LEEP was performed for those two recurrent cases. Recurrence as CIS after PDT for CIS was observed in 2 out of 7 cases (29%) 37 and 51 months later. Second PDT was performed for those two recurrent cases, resulting in CR in two cases. Recurrence as invasive cancer after PDT for CIS was observed in 2 out of 7 cases (29%) 11 and 73 months later. Operation (radical hysterectomy) was performed followed by chemotherapy and radiation. Recurrence after PDT for endocervical adenocarcinoma stage Ib1 was observed 14 months later. Operation was rejected and chemo-radiation therapy was performed for the recurrent endocervical adenocarcinoma.

Table 2. Therapy for 7 cases of Recurrence after CR

Rec rate after CR: 7／511 (1.4%)、
Time of observation: 16～234 Months
1. recurrence as SD after PDT for SD (8M, 28M later).
   2／7 (29%) → LEEP
2. recurrence as CIS after PDT for CIS (37M, 51M later).   2／7 (29%) → 2nd PDT → CR
3. recurrence as invasive cancer after PDT for CIS (11M, 73M later).
   2／7 (29%) → Ope＋Chemotherapy＋Radiation
4. rec. after PDT for EC-Adeno Ca Ib1 (14M later).
   1／7 (14%) → Chemo-radiation

Fertility Preservation after PDT for CIN3 and Early Stage Cervical Cancer

Numbers of pregnancies and deliveries after PDT were listed in the Table 3. 96 deliveries have been observed after PDT so far. Obstetrical prognosis after PDT is under continuous investigation.

Table 3. Fertility preservation after PDT for CIN3 and early stage cervical cancer

Pregnancy and delivery after PDT under continuous investigation	
Pregnancy	107 cases (139 pregnancy)
Normal vaginal delivery	75 cases
Pre-term delivery	3 cases
Caesarian section	18 cases
Artificial abortion	7 cases
Spontaneous abortion	26 cases
Ectopic pregnancy	1 case
Pregnant	9 cases

DISCUSSION

Cervical Conization (Cone Biopsy) as Standard Therapy for CIN3

Treatments for CIN include cervical cone biopsy, hysterectomy, cryotherapy, laser ablation, and Photodynamic therapy (PDT). Cervical cone biopsy enables histopathological examination of the resected specimen, whereas cryotherapy and laser ablation have the disadvantage of not allowing histological examination of the frozen or vaporized area. Although small in number, there are some patients with microinvasive or invasive cancer among those preoperatively determined to have carcinoma in situ. Cervical cone biopsy is therefore recommended for carcinoma in situ because this method allows a tissue diagnosis.

Effects of Cone Biopsy on Subsequent Pregnancy and Delivery

Recently, the effects of cone biopsy on subsequent pregnancy and delivery have attracted considerable attention. Kyrgiou et al. performed a meta-analysis of 27 studies on the obstetric prognosis following conservative treatment for CIN and early invasive cancer [2]. They found that cold knife, LEEP, and laser cone biopsy significantly increased the risk of premature birth, low birth weight, and Cesarean section.

Recurrence after Cone Biopsy

Patients with positive resection margins had a recurrence rate of 9-16% following LEEP or laser cone biopsy, whereas those with negative resection margins had a recurrence rate of 2-4% [8, 9]. Even for cases with positive resection margins, spontaneous regression was reported during the follow-up period in 61% of patients in whom the residual lesion on the uterine side was less than CIN 2 [10]. In any case, careful follow-up is needed for patients with positive resection margins. Cone biopsy should be repeated in patients with positive resection margins or recurrence [11], and hysterectomy should be considered if invasive cancer is suspected [12]. When ablation of the resection surface was performed in addition to cone biopsy, prevention of residual lesions on the uterine side and recurrence was reported.

Indication of PDT

Case which is pathologically diagnosed as CIN and early stage cervical cancer (up to stage Ia1) is a indication for gynecological PDT which is approved by the Japanese Ministry of Welfare and Labor and covered by the Japanese medical insurance. Additional indications are as follows. Case hoping preservation of fertility. Case rejecting surgical procedure such as conization. Case with high risk systemic disease which is unsuitable for conization under anesthesia. Case of old age.

Response of PDT for CIN3 and Early Stage Cervical Cancer

503 out of 520 cases (97%) of uterine cervical lesions became CR after the first PDT. 8 out of 16 PR cases became CR after second PDT. Totally, 511 out

of 520 cases (98%) became CR after PDT including second PDT. CR rates of dysplasia, CIS, and MIC, are 99%, 97%, 92%, respectively. Especially, the fact that 22 out fo 24 MIC became CR, and the rest two became PR, suggesting the efficacy of the PDT for MIC. Recurrence rate after CR is 1.4%.

Advantages of PDT

1. Cervical canal is preserved intact while cancer cells are destroyed.
2. Absolutely no bleeding during the treatment.
3. No pain, therefore, no anesthesia is needed.
4. High cure rate and low recurrence rate unlike CO2 laser vaporization.
5. No difficulties for pregnancy or delivery unlike endocervical conization.

Disadvantages of PDT

1. Photosensitivity was observed for three months after PDT.
2. Long hospitalization for three weeks was required unlike CO2 laser vaporization or endocervical conization
3. No pathological information was obtained after PDT unlike endocervical conization.

FUTURE PERSPECTIVE OF PDT IN GYNECOLOGICAL TUMORS

Soergel P assessed the feasibility and response rate of PDT with hexaminolevulinate (HAL) in cervical intraepithelial neoplasia (CIN) and human papillomavirus (HPV) infection. They concluded that HAL PDT seemed to be a non-invasive, repeatable procedure for CIN and cervical HPV infection with minimal side effects which could be easily performed on outpatient basis [14].

Soergel P also aims to evaluate the economical aspect of CIN treatment including associated pregnancy complications by comparing both methods. He concluded that for Germany, PDT has the potential to be a cost-effective treatment for high-grade CIN compared to conisation procedure. Most important, the increased perinatal morbidity, perinatal mortality and associated costs after conisation procedures are significant and may be reduced by the implementation of PDT in CIN treatment [15].

Trushina OI reported regarding PDT using Photogem or Photosens for precancer and early stages cancer of cervix uteri. Complete regression of CIN III was achieved in 50 (89%) out of 56 cases of CIN3 using PDT with Photogem. Complete regression of CIN III was achieved in 33 cases (94%) out of 35 cases of CIN3 using PDT with Photosens [16].

Istomin YP reported that PDT with the photosensitizer Photolon was applied in women of a childbearing age with CIN II and III. Complete regression of CIN II and III was achieved in 104 (92.8%) of 112 treated women [17].

We are planning to perform clinical trial of second generation PDT using small semi-conductor laser and Taraporpfin sodium (Laserphyrin) for CIN II and III in Japan (Figure 7). Taraporpfin sodium is expected to have less photosensitivity and more therapeutic effect for CIN and uterine cervical cancer than photofrin.

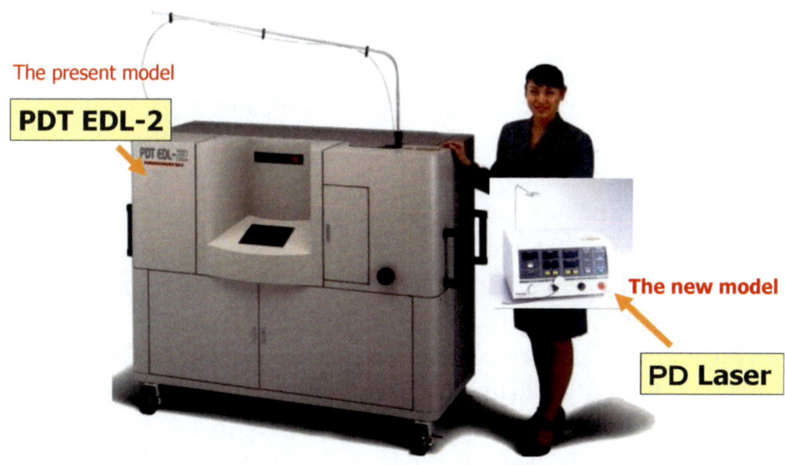

Figure 7.

CONCLUSION

Photofrin-PDT is considered to be a useful fertility preserving therapy for uterine cervical cancer up to stage Ia, which can easily be performed without bleeding, pain and anesthesia in comparison with endocervical conization.

We are planning to perform clinical trial using second generation of PDT, i.e., Laserphyrin-PDT so that we can reduce side effect of photosensitivity and admission period.

COI

Authors disclose that there are no conflicts of interests regarding this research.

ACKNOWLEDGMENTS

Authors are grateful to the Grant-in-aid from the Ministry of Health, Welfare and Labour, Ministry of Education and Science, and Sasaki Foundation.

REFERENCES

[1]   Jpn. Guideline for the treatment of cervical cancer. 2011 Edition. Edited by Japan Society of Gynecologic Oncology. Kanehara & Co., Ltd., Japan.

[2]   Kyrgiou M, Koliopoulos G, Martin-Hirsch P, ArbynM, Prendiville W, Paraskevaidis E: Obstetric outcomes after conservative treatment for intraepithelial or early invasive cervical lesions: systematic review and meta-analysis. *Lancet* 367: 489—498, 2006.

[3]   Dougherty TJ, Lawrence G, Kaufman JH, Boyle D, Weishaupt KR, Goldfarb A: Photoradiation in the treatment of recurrent breast cancer. *J Natl cancer Inst* 62: 231—237, 1979.

[4]   Hayata Y, Kato H, Konaka C, Ono J, Takizawa N: Hematoporphyrin derivative and laser photoradiation in the treatment of lung cancer. *Chest* 81: 269—277, 1982.

[5]   Muroya T, Kawasaki K, Suehiro Y, Kunugi T, Umayahara K, Akiya T, Iwabuchi H, Sakunaga H, Sakamoto M, Sugishita T, Tenjin Y: Application of PDF for uterine cerrical cancer. *Diagnostic and Therapeutic Endoscopy* 5: 183—190, 1999.

[6]   Yamaguchi S, Tsuda H, Takemori M, Nakata S, Nishimura S, Kawamura N, Hanioka K, Inoue T, Nishimura R: Photodynamic therapy for cervical intraepithelial neoplasia. *Oncology* 69 (2) : 110—116, 2005.

[7]   Sakamoto M. Safety guidelines for photodynamic therapy in the treatment of early stage cancer and dysplasia of the uterine cervix. *Laser Therapy* 21(1): 60-64, 2012.

[8]   Anderson ES, Pederson B, Nielsen K: Laser conization: the results of treatment of cervical intraepithelial neoplasia. *Gynecol Oncol* 54: 201—204, 1994.

[9]   Vedel P, Jakobsen H, Kryger-Baggesen N, Rank F, Bostofte E: Five year follow up of patients with cervical intra-epithelial neoplasia in the cone margins after conization. *Eur J Obstet Gynecol Reprod Biol* 50: 71—76, 1993.

[10] White CD, Cooper WL, Williams RR: Management of residual squamous intraepithelial lesions of the cervix after conization. *W V Med J* 89: 382—385, 1993.

[11] Ayhan A, Boynukalin FK, Guven S, Dogan NU, Esinler I, Usubutun A: Repeat LEEP conization in patients with cervical intra-epithelial neoplasia grade 3 and positive ectocervical margins. *Int J Gynaecol Obstet* 105: 14—17, 2009.

[12] Yamaguchi H, Ueda M, Kanemura M, Izuma S, Nishiyama K, Tanaka Y, Noda S: Clinical efficacy of conservative laser therapy for early-stage cervical cancer. *Int J Gynecol Cancer* 17: 455—459, 2007.

[13] Hillemanns P, Wang X, Hertel H, Andikyan V, Hillemanns M, Stepp H, Soergel P. Pharmacokinetics and selectivity of porphyrin synthesis after topical application of hexaminolevulinate in patients with cervical intraepithelial neoplasia. *Am J Obstet Gynecol.* 198(3):300.e1-7, 2008.

[14] Soergel P, Wang X, Stepp H, Hertel H, Hillemanns P. Photodynamic therapy of cervical intraepithelial neoplasia with hexaminolevulinate. *Lasers Surg Med.* 40(9):611-5, 2008.

[15] Soergel P, Makowski L, Makowski E, Schippert C, Hertel H, Hillemanns P. Treatment of high grade cervical intraepithelial neoplasia by photodynamic therapy using hexylaminolevulinate may be costeffective compared to conisation procedures due to decreased pregnancy-related morbidity. *Lasers Surg Med.* 43(7):713-20, 2011.

[16] Trushina OI, Novikova EG, Sokolov VV, Filonenko EV, Chissov VI, Vorozhtsov GN. Photodynamic therapy of virus-associated precancer and early stages cancer of cervix uteri. *Photodiagnosis Photodyn Ther.* 5(4):256-9, 2008.

[17] Istomin YP, Lapzevich TP, Chalau VN, Shliakhtsin SV, Trukhachova TV. Photodynamic therapy of cervical intraepithelial neoplasia grades II and III with Photolon. *Photodiagnosis Photodyn Ther.* 7(3):144-51, 2010.

In: Cryosurgery and Colposcopy
Editor: Lillian Watson

ISBN: 978-1-63484-507-6
© 2016 Nova Science Publishers, Inc.

Chapter 8

"THREE RINGS VULVOSCOPY": A NEW APPROACH TO THE VULVA

Vesna Harni[1,], MD, Damir Babic[2], MD, PhD, and Dubravko Barisic[3], MD, PhD*
[1]Gynecological Clinic Dr. Vesna Harni, Zagreb, Croatia
[2]University Department of Obstetrics and Gynecology, Zagreb, Croatia
[3]Department of Obstetrics and Gynecology, Villach, Austria

Keywords: colposcopy, vulva, vulvoscopy, three vulvar rings, vulvar discomfort, vulvodynia, three rings vulvoscopy

INTRODUCTION

In the attempt to colposcopically examine the vulva, it is essential to know the histology of vulvar skin, since the complexity of the vulvar anatomy requires a different assessment of the seemingly same types of lesions in this area. Thickness of the vulvar skin affects the opacity; the vascular patterns are less marked and less marked and less reliable than with colposcopy of the cervix. Vascular aberrations, such as punctuations and mosaic, can be practically seen only on the inner portions of the labia minora where the

---

[*] Corresponding address: Vesna Harni, MD, Ginekoloska poliklinika Dr. Vesna Harni, Bukovacka 1, HR-10000 Zagreb, Croatia. e–mail:vesna.harni@zg.t-com.hr.

keratin layer is thinner and vestibular epithelium does not contain a keratin layer [1].

The most recent classification of vulvar diseases by the International Society for Study of Vulvovaginal Disease (ISSVD) and the International Federation for Cervical Pathology and Colposcopy (IFCPC) from 2011 introduced a detailed description of vulvar lesions according to dermatological criteria, which includes various variables that characterize each lesion by its size, location, type, color and secondary morphology according to dermatological criteria [2, 3]. Implementation of these recommendations in daily gynecological practice results in further efforts to assess and plan the treatment of vulvar lesions.

Vulvodynia is another issue, defined as vulvar discomfort, most often described as burning pain, occuring in the absence of relevant visible finding or a specific neurological disorder, which is diagnosed using Friedrich's criteria and "per exclusion" [4–7].

Symptoms that indicate disease of the vulva include burning, stinging, soreness, irritation, feeling as if being cut with a knife or paper, stabbing, sticking, itching, inflammation and pain [8]. Very often there are no differences in symptoms between vulvar dermatosis and vulvodynia.

This was the reason for testing a new concept of vulvoscopy adapted to the anatomy of the vulva, according to the differences in histological structure and embryological origin of the vulvar structures.

THREE VULVAR RINGS

A new technique of performing vulvoscopy is proposed, taking into account three different skin types and zones that are almost ring–shaped. Instead of a random or linear vulvoscopy, this is a circular purposeful observation of the vulva, hereinafter called "Three Rings Vulvoscopy" (Figure 1). The three vulvar rings – outer, middle and inner vulvar ring are described according to hystology and embryology of the vulva.

"The Outer Vulvar Ring" includes the vulvar skin developed from the ectoderm, and it is composed of hair–bearing, keratinized skin containing sebaceous, apocrine and eccrine glands, subcutaneous fat and blood vessels, which make it a natural outer boundary of the vulva [9]. This includes the mons pubis, labia majora and the perineum.

"The Middle Vulvar Ring" encompasses the modified mucosa of the ectodermal origin, which makes an intermediate circuit between the labia majora and the vestibule. It is covered with non–hair–bearing skin, but the only appendages found are sebaceous glands, without subcutaneous fat. This includes the anterior commissure, prepuce and frenulum of the clitoris, interlabial sulci, labia minora and the fourchette.

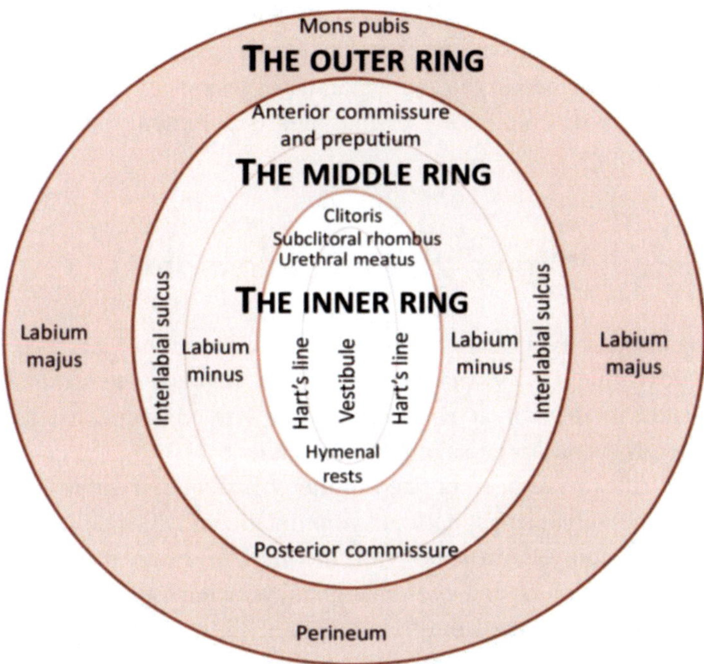

Figure 1. The three vulvar rings: outer, middle and inner vulvar ring [Reproduced from Gynaecology et Perinatology (2015), by courtesy of the authors and publisher]. The three vulvar rings are described according to histological and embryonic nature of the vulva. "The outer vulvar ring" includes the vulvar skin: the mons pubis, labia majora and the perineum. "The middle vulvar ring" encompasses the modified mucosa: the anterior commissure with the prepuce of the clitoris, interlabial sulci, labia minora and the posterior commissure (fourchette). "The inner vulvar ring" is glycogenated squamous mucosa of non–keratinized type: the clitoris, the sub–clitoral rhombus, the urethral meatus, hymenal remains, Bartholin's gland opening, Hart's line and the vestibule.

"The Inner Vulvar Ring" is glycogenated squamous mucosa of non–keratinized type, non–pigmented stratified squamous epithelium with a complete absence of skin appendages, which is of endodermal origin except for a small area immediately anterior to the urethra. This includes the clitoris, the sub–clitoral rhombus ("sulcus urethralis"), urethral meatus, hymenal remains, Bartholin's gland opening, Hart's line and the vestibule. The demarcation line between the inner and middle ring is marked by the junction of keratinized with non–keratinized epithelium on the inner aspects of the labia minora, which is referred to as the vestibular line of Hart.

The lower genital tract, in addition to the vulva, includes groins, the perianal region and the anus. The skin of the groin and perianal region is composed of the same tissue as the skin of the outer ring of the vulva and lesions may be described in the same manner as lesions of the outer ring of the vulva. Endoscopy or colposcopy of the anus is commonly known as "high–resolution anoscopy."

THREE RINGS VULVOSCOPY

During the last two years, "Three Rings Vulvoscopy" has been used in Gynecologic Clinic Dr. Vesna Harni, Zagreb (Croatia) to examine vulvar lesions related to the vulvar rings in around 400 consecutive patients with vulvar discomfort and in the asymptomatic patients [10]. In the course of this, certain regularities have been noticed in the occurrence of vulvoscopy lesions in relation to the vulvar rings, both in symptomatic and asymptomatic women.

After exclusion of patients with incomplete medical records, vulvar infection, benign tumors and pre–/malignancy, a retrospective observational study analyzed the results of the "Three Rings Vulvoscopy" in a total of 108 gynecological patients with and 108 patients without vulvar discomfort. Vulvar discomfort and colposcopic changes of the vulva were documented according to their specificity and localization using ISSVD Vulvodynia Pattern Questionnaire. In addition to the vulvoscopy, cotton–swab test, inspection of the vagina, vaginal pH measurement and microscopy of vaginal discharge were done in all patients. Based on the specificity of vulvoscopy findings, lesions were classified as "specific" and "non–specific."

"Specific lesions" were defined as the finding of eczematous inflammation with thickened, excoriated skin in lichen simplex chronicus; hypopigmented or white lesions, fusion or resorption of the labia minora and clitoral hood, loss of vulvar architecture and sclerotic changes in lichen sclerosus; white reticular pattern to extensive erosion with agglutination or resorption of the labia in lichen planus and psoriatic erythematous papules with silver, scaly plaques [11]. The diagnosis of vulvar dermatosis was confirmed histopathologically in all patients with specific lesions (n = 33).

"Non–specific findings" included non–specific erythema in the absence of infection in any part of the vulva; punctuations and papillae in the area of labia minora, Hart's line and the vestibule; the paleness and the smoothness of the sub–clitoral rhombus and the vestibule and excoriations in the absence of vulvar dermatosis [11–12].

Diagnosis of vulvodynia was based on medical history data with the determination of the index of dyspareunia, and clinical examination where signs of vulvar specific disease ("diagnosis per exclusion") were absent, in combination with positive cotton-swab test according to the actual guidelines. Non–specific findings in patients diagnosed with vulvodynia, were not relevant for the diagnosis of vulvodynia (Figure 2).

A Keyes punch biopsy was done in 21 patients with non–specific vulvoscopy finding, in all cases a specific diagnosis was excluded. Diagnostic biopsy was not performed in any asymptomatic patient, or in patients with vulvodynia and discrete skin changes not relevant for the diagnosis, following the ethical principles in the Declaration of Helsinki.

The analysis of the results of "Three Rings Vulvoscopy" revealed four groups of patients, as shown in Table 1.

Asymptomatic patients without visible vulvoscopy changes were labeled as patients with the "normal vulva."

As the previous data suggest the importance of maintaining the integrity of the barrier function of the skin to prevent the activation of inflammatory mediators on exogenous or endogenous path and psychological stress [13], we assumed that these mechanisms may play a role in the occurrence of non–specific lesions in asymptomatic patients, and named this group "impaired vulvar skin" [7].

VULVOSCOPY FINDINGS IN THE OUTER VULVAR RING

Specific vulvoscopy findings in the outer vulvar ring were present in 93.9% of patients with vulvar dermatosis. Furthermore, vulvar dermatosis was characterized by the significantly more frequent (p < 0.001) presence of specific lesions in all three vulvar ring (Figure 3).

Diagnosis of non–specific vulvoscopy findings in the outer vulvar ring was also significantly more frequent (p < 0.001) in the patients with vulvar dermatosis compared to the other groups.

Table 1. Distribution of patients depending on the symptoms and vulvoscopy findings

<table>
<tr><td colspan="5" align="center">SPECIFICITY OF VULVOSCOPY LESIONS</td></tr>
<tr><td rowspan="11">VULVAR SYMPTOMS</td><td rowspan="6">Symptomatic patients (n = 108)</td><td colspan="2">A/Specific findings (n = 33)</td><td>B/Non–specific findings (n = 75)</td></tr>
<tr><td colspan="2">VULVAR DERMATOSIS:</td><td>VULVODYNIA*</td></tr>
<tr><td></td><td>5 Lichen simplex chronicus,</td><td></td></tr>
<tr><td></td><td>23 Lichen sclerosus,</td><td></td></tr>
<tr><td></td><td>3 Lichen planus,</td><td></td></tr>
<tr><td></td><td>1 Dermatitis psoriasiformis</td><td></td></tr>
<tr><td></td><td>1 Pemphigus familiaris</td><td></td></tr>
<tr><td rowspan="2">Asymptomatic patients (n = 108)</td><td colspan="2">A/Normal findings (n = 54)</td><td>B/Non–specific findings (n = 54)</td></tr>
<tr><td colspan="2">NORMAL VULVA</td><td>IMPAIRED VULVAR SKIN</td></tr>
</table>

* = Non–specific findings in these patients were not relevant for the diagnosis of vulvodynia.

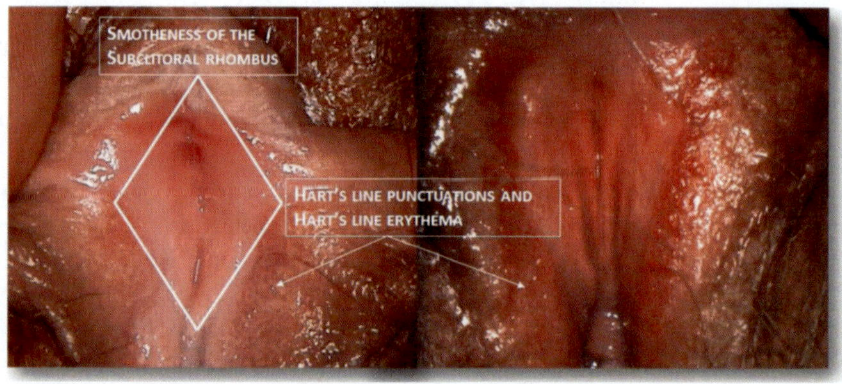

Figure 2. The smoothness of the sub–clitoral rhombus, Hart's line punctuations and Hart's line erythema in patient with vulvodynia.The smoothness of the sub–clitoral rhombus, the paleness of the urethral meatus as well as Hart's line punctuations and Hart's line papillae in the inner ring of the vulva were more often present in the patients with vulvodynia and impaired vulvar skin. Non–specific findings in patients diagnosed as vulvodynia were not relevant for the diagnosis of vulvodynia.

Non–specific findings were found in 13.3% of patients with vulvodynia and 3.7% of patients with impaired vulvar skin. These changes of the vulva in patients diagnosed as vulvodynia were not relevant for the diagnosis of vulvodynia.

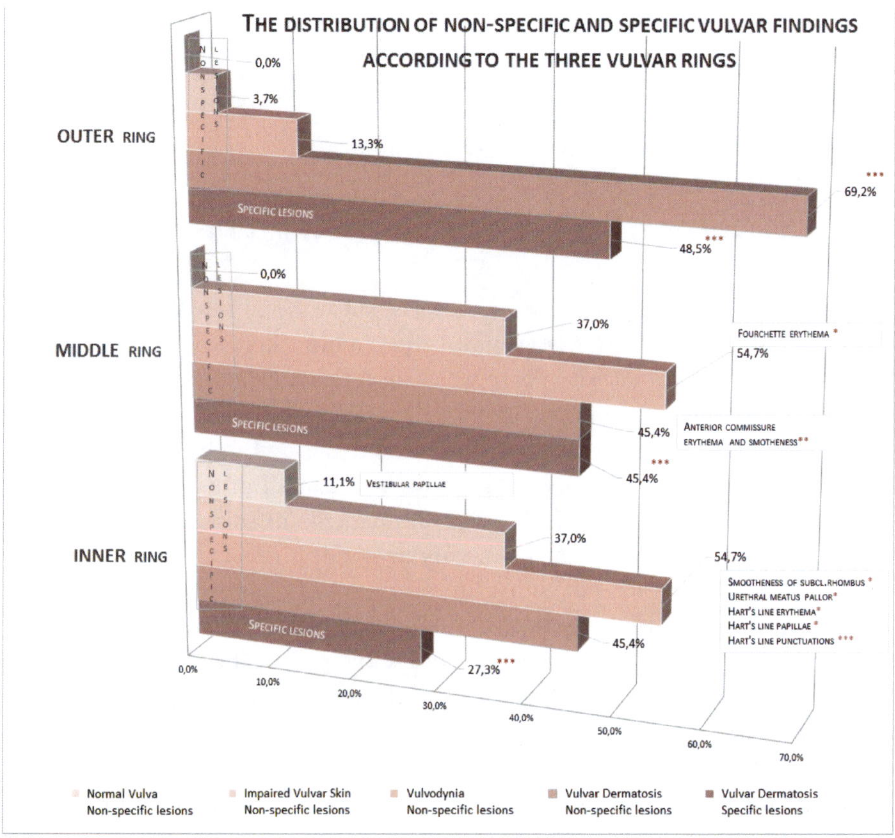

Figure 3. The distribution of non–specific and specific vulvoscopy findings according to the three vulvar rings.* = p < 0.05; ** = p < 0.01; *** = p < 0.001. Vulvar dermatosis was characterized by the significantly more frequent presence of specific lesions in all three vulvar ring. Patients with vulvodynia and impaired vulvar skin had significantly higher incidence of non–specific lesions in the inner ring of the vulva. Non–specific findings in patients diagnosed as vulvodynia were not relevant for the diagnosis of vulvodynia.

VULVOSCOPY FINDINGS IN THE MIDDLE VULVAR RING

Diagnosis of specific vulvoscopy lesions in the middle vulvar ring was significantly more frequent (p < 0.001) in the patients with vulvar dermatosis compared to the other groups.

The presence of non–specific lesions in the middle vulvar ring, specifically the erythema of interlabial sulci and the fourchette did not differ between the groups, but the incidence of the erythema (p = 0.039) and the smoothness (p = 0.019) of the anterior commissure and the prepuce, and the incidence of the excoriations in the fourchette (p < 0.001), were significantly higher in the patients with vulvar dermatosis.

VULVOSCOPY FINDINGS IN THE INNER VULVAR RING

Finding of specific lesions of the clitoris, sub–clitoral rhombus, Hart's line and in the vestibular area were significantly more likely (p < 0.001) in the group with vulvar dermatosis. There was a significant difference (p = 0.046) in the presence of any vulvoscopy findings, primarily non–specific lesions in the inner ring of the vulva in patients with vulvodynia and impaired vulvar skin compared to patients with vulvar dermatosis, and in all groups compared to a normal vulva. Non–specific findings in the patients diagnosed as vulvodynia were not relevant for the diagnosis of vulvodynia.

The smoothness of the sub–clitoral rhombus was significantly more frequent (p = 0.003) in the group of vulvodynia, whereas the paleness of the urethral meatus (p = 0.030), as well as Hart's line punctuations (p < 0.001) and Hart's line papillae (p = 0.006), were significantly higher in the groups with vulvodynia and impaired vulvar skin in relation to the vulvar dermatosis and the normal vulva.

There was no difference in the appearance of non–specific lesions of the clitoris, hymenal rests, Bartholin's gland opening and in the vestibular area between the two groups, except in relation to the normal vulva (p < 0.001).

CONCLUSION

We described an original technique for performing colposcopy of the vulva called "Three Rings Vulvoscopy", taking into account three different skin types and zones, which are approximately ring–shaped, as well as morphological evaluation of lesions according to their specificity (non–specific and specific lesions). The new vulvoscopy technique seems to be promising in the differential diagnosis of vulvar discomfort.

The vulvoscopy results suggests the importance importance of maintaining the integrity of the skin of the vulva. Vulvar care guidelines are successful for the management of vulvar complaints, and previous research has shown a decrease in mean score for dyspareunia, burning after intercourse, vulvar burning, vulvar itching and vulvar pain [4, 7, 14]. Given that the fundamental difference between the patients with vulvodynia and impaired vulvar skin is the presence of vulvar symptoms, this study could open the debate on whether the patients with impaired vulvar skin without vulvar discomfort are a possible target population for the prevention of vulvodynia.

These data raised the question whether the vulvar care measures should also be recommended to asymptomatic women with impaired vulvar skin.

"Three Rings Vulvoscopy" is being proposed in order to encourage others to adopt it and prove it in clinical practice.

Author Disclosure

Nothing to disclose.

Publishable Conflict of Interest Statement

No conflict of interest.

REFERENCES

[1]   Kesic, V. Colposcopy of the vulva, perineum and anal canal. IN Bösze P, Luesley D eds. *EAGC Course book of colposcopy*, Chapter 14; 2004; 126–63. available at: http://www.yalaphc.net/readbook/colposcopy–of–the–vulva–perineum–and–anal–canal–kntf.html. Accessed November 15, 2014.

[2]   Lynch, PJ; Moyal–Barracco, M; Scurry, J; Stockdale, C. 2011 ISSVD Terminology and Classification of Vulvar Dermatological Disorders: An Approach to Clinical Diagnosis. *J. Low Genit Tract. Dis.* 2012; 16 (4): 339–44.

[3]   Bornstein, J; Sideri, M; Tatti, S; Walker, P; Prendiville; W, Haefner, HK et al. 2011 Terminology of the Vulva of the International Federation for Cervical Pathology and Colposcopy. *J. Low Genit Tract. Dis.* 2012; 16 (3), 290-5.

[4]   Haefner, H; Collins, M; Davis, GD; Edwards, L; Foster, D; Hartmann, E et al. The Vulvodynia Guideline. *J. Low Genit Tract. Dis.* 2005; 9 (1):40–51.

[5]   Pyka, RE; Wilkinson, EJ; Friedrich, EG Jr; Croker, BP. The histopathology of vulvar vestibulitis syndrome. *Int. J. Gynecol. Pathol.* 1988; 7:249–57.

[6]   Chadha, S; Gianotten, WL; Drogendijk, AC; Weijmar Schultz, WC; Blindeman, LA; van der Meijden, WI. Histopathologic features of vulvar vestibulitis. *Int. J. Gynecol. Pathol.*1998; 17:7–11.

[7]   Petersen, E.E. Farbatlas der Vulvaerkrankungen, 3. Auflage. Kaymogyn GmbH, 2013. ISBN: 978-3-00-043086-2.

[8]   ISSVD *Vulvodynia* Pattern *Questionnaire.* Available at:https:// netforum.avectra.com/temp/ClientImages/ISSVD/3ef9c6ea-aac7-4d2b-a37f-058ef9f11a67.pdf Last accessed May 23, 2015.

[9]   Ridley's The Vulva, Third Edition. Edited by Sallie M. Neill and Fiona M. Lewis. 2009 Blackwell Publishing. ISBN: 078–1–4051–6813–7.

[10]   Harni, V; Babic, D; Barisic, D. Three Rings Vulvoscopy – A New Approach to the Vulva. *Gynaecol.Perinatol.* 2015 (in press).

[11]   Julian, TM. Vulvar Pain: Diagnoses, Evaluation, and Management. *J. Low Genit Tract. Dis.* 1997; 1 (3):185–94.

[12]   Bohm–Starke, N. Medical and physical predictors of localized provoked vulvodynia. *Acta Obstet. Gynecol.* 2010; 89:1504–10.

[13]   Slominski, A;Wortsman, J. Neuroendocrinology of the skin. *Endocr Rev* 2000; 21:457–87.

[14]   Lifits–Podorozhansky, YM; Podorozhansky, Y; Hofstetter, S; Gavard, JA. Role of Vulvar Care Guidelines in the Initial Management of Vulvar Complaints. *J. Low Genit Tract. Dis.* 2012; 16 (2):88-91.

INDEX

Q

R

S

T